Slow *But* Sure...

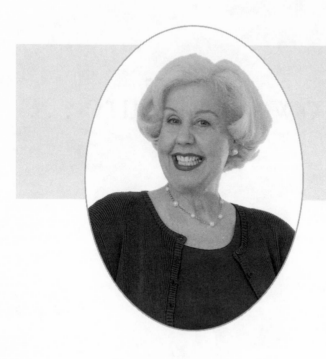

DOUBLEDAY
New York   London
Toronto   Sydney
Auckland

Slow *But* Sure...

How I Lost 170 Pounds with
the Help of God, Family,
Family Circle Magazine,
and Richard Simmons

Sandra Dalka-Prysby

Foreword by Richard Simmons

PUBLISHED BY DOUBLEDAY

a division of Random House, Inc.

1540 Broadway, New York, New York 10036

DOUBLEDAY and the portrayal of an anchor with a dolphin are
trademarks of Doubleday, a division of Random House, Inc.

Book design by Deborah Kerner

Library of Congress Cataloging-in-Publication Data

Dalka-Prysby, Sandra.
    Slow but sure: how I lost 170 pounds with the help of God,
    family, Family Circle magazine, and Richard Simmons /
    Sandra Dalka-Prysby: foreword by Richard Simmons. — 1st ed.
        p.   cm.
    1. Dalka-Prysby, Sandra—Health.   2. Overweight women—United States—
Biography.   3. Weight loss.   I. Title.
RC628.D12 1999
616.3'98'0092
[B]—DC21   98-31097
                                                                    CIP

ISBN 0-385-49217-0

March 1999

First Edition

10 9 8 7 6 5 4 3 2 1

This book is dedicated to
four incredible human beings
—Tom, Andy, Libby and Emily—
who make life worthwhile and
love more than just a word!

Why I Love Sandy

by Richard Simmons

Ring, ring, it's the telephone, and on the other end it's *Family Circle* magazine. Oh, I thought, they want to do an article on me! I was wrong, but the news was even better. They told me about a lady whose weight-loss journey was being followed up by the magazine. They had sent me the articles they had done on her. Very impressive, I thought, but there was a slight problem many of us go through called a plateau. That's why I was brought in, to evaluate this lady's eating and exercise program. My quick response was "Send her to Beverly Hills, California"—quite a ways from Beverly Hills, Michigan. "I want to meet her face-to-face."

Off on a plane she went and straight to my exercise studio, Slimmons. The lobby was very crowded and I told everyone a special guest was coming.

I waited outside and suddenly a car pulled up, the door opened (just like in the movies), and out stepped Sandy Prysby. We had never met before but I was positive this was her. The first thing I noticed was her mane of silver hair that sparkled in the sunlight as she walked toward me. Her smile made me light up. We hugged each other and I could tell she had been working out. She hugged me so hard that one of the crystal beads popped off my tank top! It was love at first squeeze. There was no time to re-create the final scene from the movie *An Affair to Remember*. We had work to do.

Before Sandy could react to all this wonder, she was meeting and greeting all my students. Many had been following her story in *Family Circle* and couldn't wait to congratulate her. I started playing my warm-up song and Sandy was right next to me. I kept my eye on her, making sure she understood the steps and what we were accomplishing in this workout. Sandy took breaks here and there but that smile got her through the whole hour.

"I've never sweat like this before," she said, all flushed and wet. Up until then Sandy had done a lot of walking, but she had never done an aerobic class like this before.

Everyone said their goodbyes because Sandy and I had to spend some time together to go over a new plan that we would create for her. Gosh, I asked Sandy so many questions. Main topics—food, her weekly exercise regimen, her husband, her children, and her goals and dreams. This was just the beginning of not a project, but a friendship. I made a file on Sandy, as I have done for thousands over the past twenty-five years. The file consisted of pictures of Sandy (full length), a fact sheet that included medical history, and food sheets, so she could write down what she was eating and I could see the rhythm of her fork. She also had to write down what exercises she had done and how much water she was drinking.

Sandy wasted no time in breaking her plateau and going for the goal. She diligently wrote me and we talked on the phone so many times. And boy, was Sandy exercising! She combined her power walking with her aerobics and toning. Every time I was in the Michigan area Sandy and her family would come see me at the mall or some personal appearance I was doing. Every time I saw her I noticed something—this wasn't the same woman who got out of the car. She was shrinking right before my very eyes. Sandy Prysby was not only a beautiful lady, but now a healthy beautiful lady.

I remember our last phone call before I sat down to write this foreword. I told her how much I loved and respected her.

"One last question before we hang up, Sandy. You've cut your weight in half. Now that's half the battle. The other half is keeping it off. Are you afraid of gaining it back?"

Without hesitating, my sweet Cinderella spoke. "I don't have that fear. I've worked very hard. I'm in better shape mentally and physically than I've ever been in my life."

Well, that's my "Love Story," and now it's time for you to fall in love with Sandy.

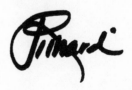

Acknowledgments

My sincere thanks go to two wonderful women—Judith Riven, my literary agent, and Judy Kern, my Doubleday editor—who know just what is needed to have dreams come true. Deep appreciation goes to two other women—Susan Kelliher Ungaro, *Family Circle* magazine's Editor in Chief, and Carla Rohlfing, Articles Editor, *Fitness* magazine—who believed I could "do it" and encouraged me on my journey. I am grateful to my WOWS ladies, especially Rhoda Kutzen and Toby Brown, who work out with me and have supported me in all my endeavors. I am thankful to my mother, Anna Marie Dalka, who learned how to help me achieve both my physical and emotional goals. I am also indebted to Muriel Wagner, R.D., who started me on my journey, and Richard Simmons, who took me to the finish line and beyond.

And, for everything, thank you, Lord!

Contents

"Slow but sure
moves the might
of the gods."

—EURIPIDES,
407 B.C.

Introduction

When is enough enough?

For me a number of things occurred in 1993 that helped me reach the point where enough was enough.

The year started the same as every new year of my adult life. I resolved to lose weight and get fit. In years past, I had failed in this resolve. This year would be different . . . it had to be different. Never before had I been this heavy—325 pounds. Never before had I smoked almost three packs of cigarettes a day. Never before had I been this close to turning fifty years of age. I was killing myself and time was running out!

I had never been slim, much less average in size. I was more than 9 pounds at birth—a hefty beginning that would prove to be a barometer of the years to come. Soon after I was born, my parents' marriage began to dissolve. My mother, overwhelmed by an impending divorce and the responsibility of two infant daughters, did what she could to handle a difficult situation. This included feeding me extra bottles of formula whenever I cried. By my first birthday I was covered with baby fat.

As the years progressed, the baby fat became just plain fat. A little con I devised as a youngster helped increase my already plump body. I would wander to nearby houses, knock on the doors, and tell the kindly neighbors how sad I was because I didn't have a daddy. Mrs. Baker was good for homemade cookies and milk. Mrs. Jackson always had ice cream with chocolate sauce, and dear, sweet Mrs. McGovern, she had everything—candy, chips, peanut butter and butter sandwiches. The only price I had to pay for these wondrous food treats was a few minutes of listening to these women's little aggravations. But the food was worth it, and I also learned to be a good listener.

My mother was frustrated with my weight. She tried to combat the fat by serving me healthy meals with lots of fruits and vegetables. She did give me sweets, but limited them to a few cookies at lunch and maybe a small bowl of ice cream at dinner. She couldn't understand why I was gaining so much weight. I, of course, kept my little forays a secret.

When I began attending elementary school, I discovered another way of getting food. While my mom packed me a small but nutritious lunch, the other kids' moms weren't as concerned about calories. The other kids had lunches loaded with food—too much food, especially cookies. I couldn't let this food go to waste. After all, there were starving children somewhere. To remedy the situation, I'd retrieve all the leftovers and, at the same time, satisfy my growing sweet tooth.

My sweet tooth as well as my appetite continued to get satisfied during my teen years. I was the neighborhood's favorite babysitter and had lots of jobs. Almost every time the parents gave

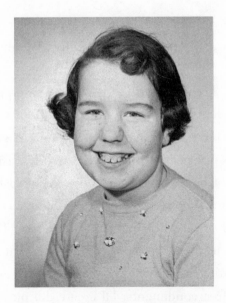

A preteen, and definitely not a beauty queen.

instructions before leaving they would add "and eat whatever you want." I did! I'd eat half of a half gallon of ice cream. Cookie crumbs were all that remained of a bag. A package of lunch meat became just a slice when I was done.

As my teen years continued, the sweet tooth combined with a desire for salt. A Coke and fries, lots of fries, was the snack of choice for all teenagers in my generation. Daily after-school trips to drive-in restaurants (your food was delivered to your car) included a couple of Cokes or sometimes a malted milk shake (vanilla, of course!) and at least one generous serving of fries. A few hours later, a large dinner topped this "snack."

This kind of eating was taking its toll. Not obese but "just overweight," I pushed into a size 16 for high school graduation. Not to worry. I was heavy, but I was also popular and had lots of friends, even boyfriends. Who cared if I was larger than most? (My mother did!) I was young and I was healthy. Weight wasn't really a problem.

In college I became even larger. I lived in an apartment with three other students, and we all took care of our own food needs. My budget was more limited than my roommates' so my "balanced meals" were lots of peanut butter sandwiches washed down with Kool-Aid, lots of boxed macaroni and cheese washed down with Kool-Aid, and, my special favorite, rice with cream of chicken soup on top, washed down with Kool-Aid, of course. (The beverage of choice because it was so inexpensive.) For lunch at the university's cafeteria, I'd order two servings of toast (four slices for 50 cents), and using the free condiments, I'd create dill pickle and mustard sandwiches. Or I'd have two orders of mashed potatoes and gravy (70 cents). These eating habits moved me up first to a size 18, then to a size 20 by college graduation.

My entry into the working world was also my passport to un-limited "good" foods. Now I had money. I had the means for morn-ing doughnuts (never just one), hamburger plates for lunch, and pizza for dinner. I also had money for the vending machines—for the 10 A.M. candy bar and the 3 P.M. candy bar(s).

During my twenties, my size 20s were getting tight. Luckily, I sewed many of my own clothes so I could fool myself about the exact size I wore. By this time I began to get worried. I wasn't concerned about my health (I was young), but I was worried about the way I looked. Although I dated, I wanted to get married, and who would want to marry a fat lady? I needed a svelte body to pursue my quest for a husband. A diet of near starvation in my late twenties brought me down to a size 14 in less than six months. I was ready!

Soon I was dating just about every Tom, Dick, and Harry in the

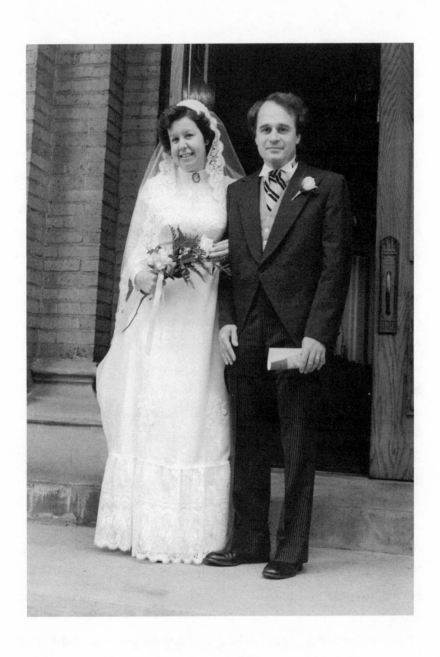

A size 16 bride, with my groom.

Detroit area. I happily settled on a Tom. After two years of dating and with my thirty-third birthday a month away, Tom and I were married in a lavish ceremony complete with the bride in a gorgeous size 16 gown. (Tom's love made me so secure that I decreased my dietary efforts and the numbers on the scale started moving back up.)

Three months into the marriage, foot surgery took me out of commission for six weeks. My wonderful husband (I did pick a good Tom!) felt sorry for me because I had to be off my feet and sedentary. His sympathy translated into a half gallon of ice cream every other day. Recovery resulted in a 30-pound weight gain and a return to size 18.

By early 1983 I was coping with three children under four years of age and this almost thirty-nine-year-old mother was overwhelmed, a word that would be part of my life for the next few years. Each time I got at least two of the kids down for a nap at the same time, I rewarded myself with a treat. My newfound "happy food" was chocolate eclairs, three at a time. Although they were expensive, I deserved them! I also learned the age-old motherly habit of "cleaning off" my children's plates. Heaven forbid I should throw any leftovers down the garbage disposal. Instead, I ate half a hot dog from one plate, the untouched spaghetti from another. I was becoming a bona fide member of the Clean Plate Club and I was expanding in the process. Size 20 clothes were getting too tight and the stretchy slacks I wore were ripping at the seams.

As my children, Andy, Libby, and Emily, grew, so did I. Fast foods accounted for much of this. Fast foods that were "necessary" because of our busy lifestyle (a soccer game here, a ballet lesson there). Convenience foods resulted in poor dietary habits for the children and more girth for me. But what was I to do? There just

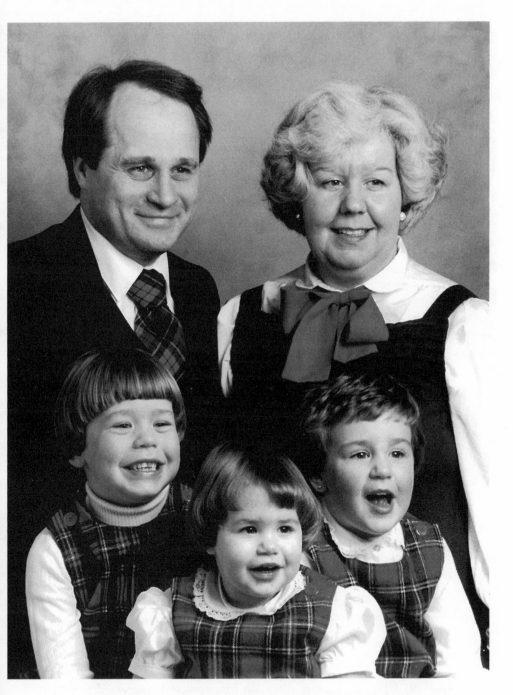

The family in October of 1984. I'm 200-plus pounds.

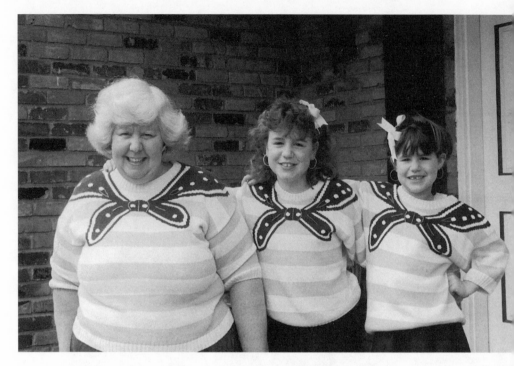

With my girls in 1990. Mom's stripes just keep on going.

wasn't time to cook. I did the best I could with such demanding schedules.

This "best" carried me over the 200-pound mark. In addition, my cholesterol was creeping up to a dangerous level (250), as was my husband's, my son's, and my youngest daughter's. But did I change our eating habits? It would take several more years and 100 more pounds for reality to hit.

Enter 1993. The number on the scale was a shock. I never, ever thought I could weigh more than 200 pounds. Now I had passed the 300-pound mark. Nor did I ever think I would wear a size 28. I had to face reality. No longer was I overweight. I was obese, an awful word in anybody's vocabulary! And, to make matters worse, I was smoking up to three packs of cigarettes a day.

Something needed to be done, and I had to do it!

On Friday, New Year's Day, 1993, I began a diet—my final attempt to realize good health. I thought I had reached the "enough is enough" point. I thought I was ready for success.

I was wrong. In the weeks that followed I goofed so many times that I spent the first few months of the year riddled with guilt. I did manage to take off, put on, and take off 15 pounds, but it wasn't easy. It was the same old battle I had fought for years, I was discouraged. I thought this time would be different.

By May 1993, I was 310 pounds and extremely depressed. In a few weeks we would be taking a family trip to Washington, D.C. How could I walk around the nation's capital and visit all the monuments? My excess weight was restricting my movements in our own home. It would wreck the family's vacation!

My 160-pound husband told me not to worry. He would take the children sight-seeing. I could relax, he said. But I didn't. How had I reached the point where I could no longer share things with my family? What kind of wife and mother was I?

Sight-seeing wasn't my only concern about going to Washington. While there, we would be staying with a former boyfriend of mine. We hadn't seen each other for years (I was under 200 pounds at our last meeting) and I was embarrassed. What would he think of me? Why did I get so fat?

The other concern involved my son, a wonderful then-thirteen-year-old. Our trip was planned around his Odyssey of the Mind world competition at the University of Maryland. I had coached his seven-member team and it had a good chance to win the finals. If they won, I would have to accompany the team up onstage to accept the award before an audience of thousands. (I wasn't sure I could even climb the steps to the stage.) I didn't want my son to be ashamed of me. I even thought of saying a prayer that the team wouldn't win. Now I really felt guilty! How could I have done this (gained so much weight) to myself and to my children, my wonderful children?

As the vacation drew closer, my questions multiplied. "Why?" "Why?" "Why?" The one question that kept coming to the forefront was "Why can't I lose weight?" I needed an answer, but, more important, I needed to dig deep inside myself and find the commitment, the strength, the motivation to succeed. I knew I needed to lose weight; I wanted to lose weight, but did I really want to do what was necessary to achieve this goal?

For the rest of the month, I spent some time each day concentrating on my strengths and asking God for help. Many times a day I looked at myself in the mirror and said out loud that I was worth good health. I worked on liking myself and, by taking a little time, I discovered that I not only liked myself, but I also loved my essence—that specialness that is me alone. (I continue these rituals daily and believe these efforts are what keeps the motivation in place.)

I dug deep inside myself and eliminated all the excuses ("my child is sick," "my husband lost his job," "my mother doesn't understand," "my children weren't good today," "I'm tired," and a million more) that had resulted in past diet failures. Instead, I concentrated on past successes and reviewed what it had taken to succeed.

Could I do it again? Could I lose weight finally and forever?

One day I awoke with such positive feelings that it was almost as if I had been "touched by an angel." (Too bad it wasn't the "fat fairy"—you know, the one with the magic wand who takes away all the fat while you're sleeping! The one who had never visited my house, but whom I continued to dream about and wish for . . . that is, until this day!) For whatever reason, when I awoke on May 26, 1993, I knew totally and deeply that I had reached the point where enough was enough. Also, I knew—deep down—that I would succeed. Slowly but surely I would lose weight and get fit.

But how?

I decided to seek help from my family and friends. I also decided to take a really big step and ask *Family Circle* magazine for help. That very morning I wrote to the editors of this popular women's magazine and made the following suggestion:

> *I propose that* Family Circle *help a forty-eight-year-old mother of three children save her life. The woman, an active and popular suburban at-home mom, is 150 pounds over-weight and smokes up to three packs of cigarettes a day. She has spent more than thirty-five years on reducing diets— some successful for a while, some not. She has also tried for five years to give up smoking.*
>
> *This woman is one and a half years away from her fiftieth birthday and knows if she doesn't do something now, she may not have another chance. She needs help to accomplish this major project. I propose that* Family Circle *provide her with a nutritionist, a diet plan, a smoke-ending program, and, more important, a medium to tell her story and struggles and provide her with someone (your readers) to whom she's accountable.*
>
> *This woman wants to lose weight and give up smoking for herself. She wants to feel, look, and be healthy so that she can live a long life and enjoy her family.*

I am this woman. I am the one who needs help, and I'm desperate.

Family Circle agreed to help. The magazine would pay for a nutritionist, who could also help eliminate the cigarettes, and I would share my challenge with its readers. It would take a few months to get everything in place. In the meantime, I stayed at 310 pounds. I ate and decided to wait.

I started my program in September 1993 and in January 1994 the magazine announced my 150-pound-weight-loss goal, complete with a photo of me in a leotard and tights. I was exposed. I was now "public." There was no turning back. I had to succeed, and I would!

Over the past five years *Family Circle*'s readers have followed my progress. Viewers have seen me on *The Maury Povich Show* and other national television shows. Both readers and viewers have learned how Richard Simmons, one of the world's best fitness experts and motivators, has joined me, thanks to *Family Circle,* in my quest for success. He's helped me get to the finish line (and past it) and he's helping me keep the weight off.

I've lost 170 pounds, and because I followed a "slow but sure" philosophy, I've changed my whole life and lifestyle.

You, too, can change your lifestyle and, in turn, your life. This book will help you to achieve your own success in losing weight and getting fit. It contains my journal notes, lots of tips that have enabled me to reach success, and the knowledge that I have acquired during the past five years.

I didn't achieve this weight loss without a struggle. Experts didn't do it all for me. I worked very hard not to eat the pizza that my three teenagers brought into the house. It was especially hard to be "good" when my husband lost still another job during my

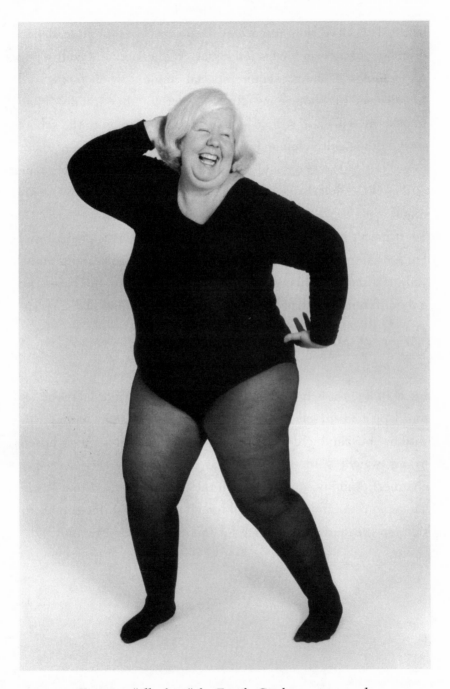

Exposing "all of me" for Family Circle at 310 pounds.

battle. (We have now discovered he has severe attention deficit disorder, the reason for his job losses. Medication and counseling are helping.) I had to acquire special stamina when family and friends tried to sabotage my efforts (something they still do). I had to push myself—and still do—out of the house to go to the school track or the health club and walk three or four miles a day . . . or to get out of the chair and pop a Richard Simmons aerobic tape into my VCR and dance and stretch for forty minutes in my family room.

It hasn't been easy, but getting healthy and fit is doable. And I'm no different from you. I'm just your average wife and mother, your next-door neighbor, with all the same problems you have. The only difference is that I have learned, with a slow but sure approach, how to lose weight and get fit.

If I can do it, so can you!

Incidentally, the whole family had a wonderful time in Washington. I pushed myself and went on some of the sight-seeing trips with my husband and kids. The old boyfriend, although surprised by my weight gain, said I was as charming as ever (he's the charmer). And my son's team won the Odyssey of the Mind World Championship and I made it, although slowly, with my son at my side, up the steps to the stage for the awards presentation.

Chapter 1

Enough Already!

How do we reach the point where enough is enough? How do we get to that place deep down inside of us that pushes us to action?

It would be nice if one day all of us overweight individuals—that's 40 percent of the population—woke up and realized that our health, and in fact our very lives, was being impacted by the extra pounds, the poor eating habits, the inactivity. But that's usually not how it happens. Sure, we know that being overweight is unhealthy. We're constantly bombarded by the media with talk about the dangers of too much fat, too little exercise, too many pounds. But having all this information usually doesn't make us do anything.

It's looking in the mirror, too tight clothes, the number on the scale, the special events—a child's wedding, an "over the hill" birthday, a class reunion—or even a small thing like having difficulty tying our shoelaces that spurs us on to action. We finally decide "once and for all" to rid ourselves of the pounds. Unfortunately, the action we take isn't always the best.

In our quest to lose weight we turn to fast solutions, "miracle" diets that guarantee success. We spend money, lots of money, at diet centers that put us on starvation programs—fewer than 1,000 calories a day. We turn to doctors who willingly agree to prescribe that new pill or encourage us into a surgical room for stapling or tying or making small balloons out of our stomachs. We drink protein liquids and forgo food. We eat cabbage soup and a few other things for seven days. We drink two gallons of water a day to flush out massive amounts of such proteins as lean meats, fowl, fish, cottage cheese, and eggs to slim down. We eat ice cream—French vanilla is best—and beets for three days for a "guaranteed" 10-pound weight loss. We have hot dogs, bananas, eggs, and nothing else, to push the numbers down the scale. We look everywhere for the answer to years of abusing our bodies. And although we want the answers, we want fast results with a minimal amount of effort. (Yay! A new diet promises 15 pounds off in a week by eating everything we want and no exercise. Yep! That's for us!)

So we start and we fail. Maybe enough wasn't enough.

But it was! Anytime we reach the point of desperation, the point where we not only want to lose weight and need to lose weight, but we decide we *can* lose weight, *we can do it*. However, it's at this point that we need to know—safe and effectively—*how* to lose weight.

One thing we don't need is a diet. *A diet is something we do to lose weight as fast as we can so we can go back to eating the way we did before!* Where does that get us? As soon as the diet is over, we begin to put the pounds back on. We go back to the same bad eating habits and make the same mistakes as before the diet.

What we need is a lifestyle change—a way of living with foods, all kinds of foods, that works. And we need exercise, a regular and realistic exercise program that does not just provide a temporary fix but becomes a lifelong healthy habit no matter our age. (Researchers are finding increasing evidence that a healthy diet and regular exercise are the best antidotes to aging—and it's never too late to start.)

Although we know the benefits of exercise, oftentimes we forget about this important aspect of a successful weight-loss program. A healthy food plan and a good exercise program must go hand in hand, or make that "foot in foot," if we are to reach our goals.

It helped me, and it can help you, to visualize your weight-loss challenge as a road—a road that ends at a healthy weight and good fitness. See yourself slim, fit, and happy at the end of this road to good health. The road you visualize may span just a short distance, reflecting your need to lose 20 or 30 pounds. Or your road may be longer, much longer, if you need to lose 100 or more pounds. No matter the distance, with patience and persistence, it's a journey that can be completed.

Many of us have traveled this road, but most of us have never gone the distance. We've stopped before reaching the end, before reaching our goal. Maybe the reason for not achieving success is that we traveled this road by dieting alone. We didn't add exercise to our travel plans.

Visualize yourself at the beginning of the road. You're pumped up. You're excited. You're ready!

You start your diet. It's going to take you to the end of the road. But dieting alone is like hopping on one foot. You start the journey, hopping and hopping and hopping. Soon you're exhausted. You don't get very far. It's difficult to hop on one foot. You give up the trip.

This time will be different. This time you will add exercise. That's what I did.

Now picture this. Consider diet one of your legs, exercise the other. You have to use both feet to complete your journey. With two feet and a slow but sure pace, you can reach your goal. You might get a little tired once in a while and you may even go off the road, but you'll have two feet to get you right back on track.

Close your eyes and see yourself at the beginning of the road. Look down at your two feet. (In your mental picture make sure you have athletic shoes on your feet. You're going to need them for your journey.) Now raise your head and see yourself down at the end of the road. See yourself reaching your goal. See the big smile on your face.

Slow but sure. That's how I reached my goal. And all the while I was on the road, a very long road marking 170 pounds, I saw myself reaching the end. I knew I would do it from the start. That's because this time I added the second foot. I added exercise. And I added visualization. Visualization, combined with the conviction that enough was enough.

Here's another visualization exercise that worked for me. Picture your excess weight as a mountain of fat. This mountain grew a little at a time—five pounds one year, three pounds another—until now it seems enormous in size. In your mind, put yourself on top of this mountain. Really look at yourself. You're probably not very happy. You don't like where you are and you want to get down from this mountain as soon as possible.

We all have a tendency to want what we want *now*. And weight loss is no exception. We want the weight off *now!* This is why we turn to the quick fixes, the crash diets. But these can be dangerous, especially when you're on top of a mountain. Think about it.

If you descend a mountain too fast, there's the possibility that you'll slip and fall and hurt yourself. Consider those times when you've tried to run down a small hill. You started off in a frenzy of delight, but as the momentum built, you probably felt you were losing control, and maybe you even did. It's easy to fall when you're going too fast and lose control. Now imagine what it would be like running down a giant mountain of fat. The danger of falling is even more likely.

The only safe way to descend from your mountain of fat is one step at a time (wearing the proper athletic shoes, of course!). Visualize yourself descending this mountain using good food and exercise as your tools. See yourself safely accomplishing the descent slowly and on solid footing. Down, down, down. It's not a straight downward journey. This mountain of fat wasn't created all at once. The pounds of weight were gained in stages over the years, forming plateaus along the way. These plateaus are still there and you'll reach them on the downward journey.

This time, on this journey, when you reach a plateau, don't get discouraged. This time when you reach a plateau, enjoy the view. Remember where you started and praise yourself for your success, no matter how short the descent. Fortify yourself with healthy nourishment and regular exercise so that you will have the stamina to complete the journey when you get off the plateau. Visualize yourself enjoying the view and continuing with your fitness program each time you reach another plateau.

Forming a mental picture of successfully completing your weight-loss goal is a positive way to stay motivated and focused. In past weight-loss attempts, I didn't make use of visualization. Instead, I did what I know now were negative things. Once I made a small cow out of felt material to hang on the refrigerator. On it I put the words HOLY COW! ARE YOU EATING AGAIN? It was meant to keep me out of the refrigerator. It didn't! It just informed everyone who visited my kitchen that I had an eating problem.

Another time it was a picture of a pig, a gigantic pig, that I hung on the refrigerator. (I sure thought well of myself at that time!) I even had the fortitude (or insanity) to put a photo of myself, complete with bulges and rolls of fat visible beneath and around my bathing suit, on the refrigerator. (What would heavy people do without a refrigerator?) This extremely unflattering photo didn't stop me from eating, but it did keep my family members out of the kitchen. I think they lost their appetite whenever they saw it!

Enough already! Why do we do these things to ourselves? Why do we choose the negative when the positive can be so much more rewarding?

When enough is really enough, and you'll know when this is, a healthy food plan (you might consider the one I followed, but check with your doctor first!) and a realistic exercise program, combined with *positive visualization,* can work. It did for me.

I exchanged visual aids (they didn't work anyway) for visualization. I formed mental pictures of the slim person I planned to be, the one I knew I could be. I concentrated on these mental images on a regular basis. For five years I "saw" the woman I am today.

One visualization effort I combined with reality. At the beginning of my journey, I purchased a very sexy negligee in a medium size and hung it on a hook on the back of the bathroom door. Every day when I looked at this lovely gown, I saw myself wearing it. Now I am!

Tips for Staying Motivated

1. Love yourself. Make a list of all your gifts, your beauty, your strengths. Hang this list on your mirror or the refrigerator or any other place where you can see it daily. Read it daily . . . and believe it!

2. Replace negative images and thoughts with positive ones. Create a visual picture of a healthy, fit you—the person you're becoming. Push this positive picture of yourself to the front of your mind whenever you feel discouraged.

3. Take time—even if it's only ten minutes—each and every day for complete privacy to focus your thoughts on yourself and your fitness program. Use this time to remind yourself that you are being and will continue to be successful. Use this time to renew your determination.

4. Draw up a contract with yourself stating that you're committed to a healthy lifestyle. List realistic ways (including a good food plan and exercise program) you are going to fulfill your contract. Determine doable goals. Keep this contract in an accessible place, e.g. your nightstand, so you can review it periodically.

5. Solve problems as they occur, otherwise they can impede your progress. If you resolve stressful situations when they arise, they won't become excuses to lead you away from your goals.

6. Review your obligations and discard those that are not good for you. You need time to get and stay healthy; you don't need to be saddled with activities that don't bring rewards.

7. Rid yourself of negative "friends"—those who do not believe that you can be successful. Instead, reach out to one or two individuals who will support you and help you.

8. Believe in yourself. Don't concentrate on past failures, but on all your successes—no matter how small—in all areas of your life.

9. Ask for loving help from your family. Tell them what you want to accomplish and how they can help, e.g. by refraining from bringing unhealthy food into the house, freeing up your time so you can exercise, encouraging you with positive messages, etc.

10. Seek God's help! I do every day and He has been there for me every step of the way!

ALWAYS REMEMBER . . . YOU ARE WORTH IT! YOU ARE WORTHY OF SUCCESS! AND YOU WILL SUCCEED!

Chapter 2

A Practice Run!

After the editors of *Family Circle* magazine agreed to help with my "get fit, get healthy" program, I was assigned two tasks. I needed to find a nutritionist in my area who would guide me in a sensible weight-loss program, someone who would also encourage me in my efforts to end cigarette smoking. And I was to keep a journal of my progress, struggles, and feelings.

AUGUST 23, 1993 (FIRST JOURNAL ENTRY)
I started the week in a depressed state. Just a few weeks to go before starting a "new way of living." I do so much want to be healthy and feel good, but at the same time, I feel a loss . . . a loss of a lifestyle I've become accustomed to. It may not be a healthy lifestyle, but it's familiar . . . it's cigarettes, it's my comfortable leather chair (the one I sit in much too often), and it's all the food I eat without ever giving much thought to what it is or what it is doing to my body. All these things have taken a toll on me. I now weigh 300-plus pounds!

Although I have firmly and passionately decided that I must change my lifestyle . . . I must get healthy (or I will die early), I still feel somewhat sad at leaving what has been. I am also a little afraid of what will be!

Then I look at my husband—a truly good man—and our three beautiful children. I like being with my family. I want to be with them as long as possible. I want to participate totally in all the fun activities we do. I don't want to run out of breath from smoking or the excess pounds. I want to eliminate the restraints that have made me a passive participant.

I want all this, I want to succeed, but I'm afraid of starting this journey. In a few weeks the trip begins!

Thursday, August 26, 1993

Today was dismal! I met with the head of Preventive and Nutritional Medicine at the major hospital in my area to discuss working with him on a healthy weight-loss program. I told him I needed a balanced food program that I and the readers of Family Circle could follow. He pushed fasting because was so heavy. He did, after much bullying on his part, offer a food plan of fish, fowl, and vegetables for a year—no fruits, no breads, no fats, nothing else. I knew I would never be successful on such a program. It was too restrictive, too unrealistic.

This "helper of the overweight" also asked, if I was so determined to lose weight, why was I so large, and after looking me up and down, he said, "I'll bet you're a good cook!" I left his office in tears.

Friday, August 27, 1993

What a difference twenty-four hours make! I found a nutritionist to work with today. She's Muriel G. Wagner, a registered dietitian and a charter fellow of the American Dietetic Association. In addition, she has a Ph.D. in counseling, just what I need!

Dr. Wagner believes in working with food to develop a new life-style—a new way of living! She follows the guidelines of such respected groups as the American Heart Association and the Department of Agriculture.

In addition to being a pleasant, warm, and optimistic person, Dr. Wagner calls her clients nightly to help them plan their menu for the next day. She wants me to "think" about what I am going to eat. Studies indicate, according to her, that individuals who write down the food they plan to eat have a much better success rate in achieving their weight-loss goals.

That night as I was thinking about Dr. Wagner's approach—the nightly food planning—a light went on in my head. Of course! We never go on a trip without first mapping it out, an architect never puts up a building without first drawing up plans, a seamstress never makes a dress without having a pattern. It makes sense to plan what I am going to eat. I've gained weight by putting things in my mouth without thinking. Now let's try thinking!

WEDNESDAY, SEPTEMBER 1, 1993
My first day as a nonsmoker. (Dr. Wagner suggested that I first give up smoking; the weight-loss program will follow in two weeks.) What a rough day. I have one of those patches on, but it doesn't seem to help the habit part of smoking. I spent a lot of time today in the bathtub and in bed, two places I never smoke. And I went to church (I don't smoke there either) and prayed to God for help. At this rate I'll be clean, well rested, and holy! It's going to be hard, but I'll continue to grit my teeth (at least that way I can't shove a cigarette into my mouth)!

WEDNESDAY, SEPTEMBER 8, 1993
My first official meeting with Dr. Wagner. She weighed me (310 pounds) and she took my measurements (I'm a 54-50-57½ babe!). She put me on an 1,800-calorie, balanced food plan and suggested that I start walking each and every day with an eventual goal of three miles a day in forty-five minutes.

The food plan I was first placed on included eleven servings from the bread group, 10 ounces from the meat group, two servings of milk/dairy products, three fruits, two fat servings, and unlimited vegetables. This, to me, was a lot of food. I couldn't believe I would lose weight on this food plan.

The plan served me well at the start of my program and resulted in an 80-pound weight loss in less than two years. However, after a depressing six-month stall, Richard Simmons entered my life in March 1996, thanks to *Family Circle* and a letter from me. He altered the food plan—reduced the breads and proteins and limited the vegetables. And he cut my caloric intake to 1,500 calories a day.

I was lucky. I had a nutritionist and the nation's leading diet guru to help assure my success. However, I discovered that it was *me* who did all the work . . . made the choices . . . kept the commitment! You don't need experts to be successful. You can do it—lose weight and get healthy—yourself! All you need is determination and the proven information (it worked for me!) found throughout this book. And you need to move your feet more than your fork!

THE FIRST WEEK ON THE PLAN, SEPTEMBER 12–17, 1993
Each and every day began with prayers. Then I followed the food plan exactly. I even ate breakfast for the first time in years. (Skim

milk, yuck!) *My former breakfast had consisted of a few diet colas and lots of cigarettes. Now, each and every day I feel full. I'm not even afraid of weekends anymore. There's lots of food and variety on this program. I know this food plan is definitely doable!*

WEDNESDAY, SEPTEMBER 22, 1993
I didn't go to Libby's open house at school because I can't fit into the desks. I'm lucky I have a trim (and willing) husband. Tom went. Next year I'll be able to go to all the kids' functions!

FRIDAY, SEPTEMBER 24, 1993
I have followed the food plan perfectly, but I don't think I've lost much weight. Dr. Wagner won't let me get on the scale. She says the scale can hamper progress. According to her, if you cheat on the food plan and still lose weight, you'll be tempted to continue to cheat. On the other hand, if you follow the food plan exactly, but you don't lose as much weight as you think you should, you will become discouraged. In either case, getting on the scale proves to be negative.

FRIDAY, OCTOBER 1, 1993
My sixteenth wedding anniversary. Most of my married life—and my single life, too—I've been overweight and unhealthy. Now I'm tired of dragging around this extra poundage . . . and I'm tired of not feeling sexy and feminine, especially around my husband. Tom is always willing, but I always decline. I just can't. I look in the mirror and I'm disgusted with what I see. My fat is preventing me and my husband from enjoying one of the benefits of love and marriage. We haven't had sex for three years. I'm lucky Tom hasn't had an affair! On this anniversary I vow that Tom and I will have a whole marriage by this time next year.

FRIDAY, OCTOBER 8, 1993

I confessed to Dr. Wagner that I wasn't measuring or weighing my food (a must for success!). I eyeball everything and I know that my eyes see gigantic halves of cups. I promise to improve on this . . . it's just laziness. One thing I'm not lazy about is my walking. I'm now up to a rather fast mile and a half daily. My friend Mary Sue Lanigan calls me daily and gets me out. I'm no longer the Beverly Hills (Michigan) slug!

SUNDAY, OCTOBER 24, 1993

I went to church today. I don't like sitting in the pews. I can't kneel when everybody else does, so we sit in back on the chairs. Luckily, the church has purchased new and sturdier chairs. An old chair caused me an embarrassing situation a few years ago. I was sitting on one of the old chairs and had just returned from communion. "Please, dear God, help me lose weight," I prayed. Then it happened. The chair broke and I fell to the floor. My dress flew up. My arms and legs went in all directions. Everyone gasped. My children and husband rushed to my aid. Tom tried to help me up, but I was dead weight. Then some men offered to help. That made it worse. They couldn't get me up. I yelled, "I can get up myself." They backed away. I got on my knees, then, with the aid of another chair, I forced myself—red face and all— up. I felt so small because I was so large.

SUNDAY, OCTOBER 31, 1993 (HALLOWEEN)

I am really proud of myself. For more than a week I had Snickers candy bars in the house to pass out tonight, and I didn't sneak one, not one! Notice the word I used, "sneak." That's a favorite word of fat people. We "sneak" because we know we shouldn't have such foods as pizza, candy, ice cream, etc. But yay! Success. No sneaking; no Snickers!

Although I "did good" with the Halloween candy—I didn't even rummage through the kids' bags—I learned as I got further into my program that there are better ways to approach special occasions and situations. The secret: PLANNING and CREATIVE THINKING.

Now I plan for events by coming up with alternatives to unhealthy foods. I think of ways to keep the festiveness in and the temptations out.

For Halloween, I pass out pencils, gift certificates, coins, and other nonfood items. For Valentine's Day and Easter, I limit candy and give Andy, Libby, and Emily small gifts, such as CDs, beauty supplies, sporting goods, clothing. For Christmas, we forgo a whole day of baking and eating cookies. We make less tempting pumpkin bread instead. (This baking switch has enabled us to create a new tradition for the family. It takes only a few hours to bake pumpkin bread, so we use the remaining time to go to a church and help make the food and feed the hungry in Detroit's inner city.)

WEDNESDAY, NOVEMBER 3, 1993 (MY BIRTHDAY)
I'm forty-nine years old today and I'm mad. I don't mind my age. What I do mind is that no member of my family even wished me happy birthday when they left today. So what did I do? I went to the Sara Lee Outlet, got a free birthday cake, and ate the whole thing! I thought I deserved it. I thought it would taste good, but all it did was make me feel guilty. I ended the day with prayers and some deep thoughts, and, in the process, I learned something. The birthday cake feast pointed out that I have to stay away from "good excuses" if

I'm to be successful. I can't let anger, stress, other people's actions, and other such factors keep me from completing my journey. I vowed to be more aware of why I eat unhealthy foods, and to plan better for these situations.

Why We Eat!

We eat because we're hungry, but that's not the only reason we eat. Many times we eat because we're bored, or as a substitute for love and friendship, or we have a problem, or because we're depressed or stressed. Other times we eat just because the food is there in our cupboards (or in restaurants, in vending machines, or a phone call and free delivery away).

Sometimes we eat because the food looked good on a TV commercial or in a magazine advertisement. Or because a friend or family member raved about how good it tasted.

We also eat certain foods because we like them. Or someone offered them to us and we couldn't refuse. (We didn't want to hurt the giver's feelings!) We eat certain foods because we're hungry and there's nothing else available, or we don't have time to prepare anything else, or it was the only food we could afford.

If we know why we eat and if we do a better job of planning what we eat, we will be more successful in reaching our goals. This means having the right foods on hand and the wrong foods out of sight and, therefore, out of mind.

MONDAY, NOVEMBER 8, 1993
I have not been feeling well for the past few weeks so I saw the doctor today. I have pneumonia and, in addition to medicine, I was put on lots of liquids and lots of rest. I'm not going to worry about my food plan or exercise. I'll just work toward getting healthy.

THURSDAY, NOVEMBER 25, 1993 (THANKSGIVING)

Aside from pumpkin pie (minus crust), I ate just what I was supposed to eat today. Sure, maybe I ate a little more turkey than allowed, but basically I followed the food plan.

I am still sick. I am tired of coughing and trying to catch my breath.

FRIDAY, DECEMBER 3, 1993

Although I can't seem to get well and I should have stayed home and in bed, Tom and I went to a Christmas party. I wore a new outfit that looked great on me. But there was a problem. Earlier in the day I bought the largest-sized panty hose available at the store, but they weren't large enough. They only came up to my hips. I didn't have time to get other hose so I had to wear them. First I put on a pair of underpants, then the panty hose, then another pair of underpants so the hose wouldn't fall down. The hose were extremely tight around my hips, so tight that they made an indentation that could be seen through my clothes. I didn't want to dance with Tom because I thought everyone at the party could see the line made by the indentation. Tom was upset. He loves to dance and he was looking forward to dancing with me tonight. I couldn't have danced even if there wasn't a line. The panty hose were so small they squeezed my thighs together and within a short period of time, my thighs were painfully chapped. I was miserable. I hate being fat!

SATURDAY, DECEMBER 11, 1993

After a trip to the hospital emergency room because of breathing problems, I spent the rest of the day in bed. The medicine and the illness are making me depressed. And I'm especially upset because I can't concentrate on my food plan, and exercise is totally out of the question. I'm too sick!

I've always tried to be an optimistic person about everything, even my extra weight. But I'm losing it! I need to get well so that I can be active. I'll never lose weight—or feel physically fit—without exercise. I want to be a success. I'm tired of being fat. It's like being dragged down by a horseback rider—and I'm the horse! Imagine carrying a person who weighs 150 pounds around on your back all the time. You can never put this person down. You always have to carry this person around. You have to walk with this person . . . shop with this person . . . cook with this person . . . clean with this person. That's how I feel. I want to get this person off my back. It's hard to carry around 150 extra pounds. Losing my excess weight—the "person" I'm carrying around—is going to be like being granted freedom. I can hardly wait!

DECEMBER 13–15, 1993 (IN NEW YORK, NEW YORK)
Tom, the kids, and I are in New York to tape The Maury Povich Show. *What an experience. It's not easy to bare your soul on national TV. But maybe my struggle and my family's concern will help others. It was especially hard because I still feel so lousy.*

While in New York, we did a lot of walking. For me walking is a chore because of my weight, and now because of my illness. My husband and the kids walked too fast for me. I was always steps, sometimes blocks, behind. I looked up ahead and saw my family laughing and talking together. I was too far behind to hear what they were saying. I was left out, although not on purpose. It was because I'm so fat that I can't keep up with them. If they knew how hurt I am at times like this, they would feel really bad. But it's not their fault. Sometimes I yelled for them to wait up, but most times I didn't. I hated to draw attention to the fact that I was so far behind. It only pointed out how overweight I really am!

While walking around New York was difficult on me, so were

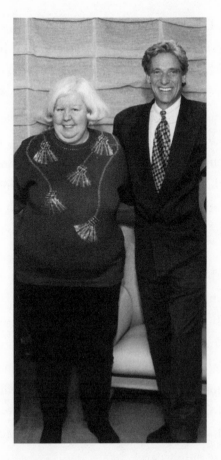

With Maury Povich before my first appearance on his show.

taxi rides. I always seemed to be on the wrong side of the taxi when we arrived at our destination. Tom and the kids would pop out of their door while I had to shove my ample body from one side of the cab to the other. It took a lot of effort and a lot of time to do this. I was embarrassed and I worried that the driver would add extra charges for the amount of time it took me to get out of the cab.

SATURDAY, DECEMBER 18, 1993

Although I undertook this program so that I would be healthy, I also want to look good. Even though I have been overweight much of my life, I have always felt that I am a beauty who needs to be discovered. I want to know what it is like to be skinny, or at least at my desired weight. But the thought of this scares me at times. I have read that research shows that heavy individuals, especially women, are the happiest. And I have always been happy. This is why I have so many friends. I'm fun to be around. I want desperately to lose weight, but what if I lose my good personality in the process?

Soon after the above journal entry—December 23, to be exact—I was admitted to the hospital. My illness had reached the critical stage. The idea of spending the holidays confined in a hospital depressed me.

I was hospitalized for six days. Family and friends visited often, bringing with them an enormous number of unhealthy food treats. They felt sorry for me. Because I felt sorry for myself, I ate everything that was brought to me, and with relish! My food plan was placed on hold. I didn't care!

When I returned home, the food gifts continued. My recovery was marked by rest and eating, eating and rest. It would be weeks before I had the energy and desire to start my weight-loss/fitness journey again.

Chapter 3

Okay, Now!
Let's Get Serious!

It was January 1994. The commitment, the food plan, the exercise, all went by the wayside, more specifically, roadside—remember that road to good health and fitness—for valid reasons. (In addition to illness, my start was delayed by the death of my mother-in-law, my husband losing still another job, the stress of the holidays, and a number of major and minor annoyances.) These kept me at the beginning of the road. Very little progress was made.

However, now—at the start of yet another new year—it was time to get, and stay, serious. No more excuses. I was turning fifty years of age in November. If I was going to do it, the time was now!

I decided to concentrate first on my food plan and eating correctly. (Exercise would have to wait for a few weeks anyway. Although my health had improved, my lung capacity wasn't up to 100 percent.) So I started the year focused on healthy foods and healthy eating. I read articles, asked questions, did research. I wanted the knowledge to be successful. I made it my goal to become an expert. I no longer wanted to be a passive participant in my life. I decided to be actively involved in my success.

At the same time I was reading and doing research into healthy eating, I was preparing to earnestly and faithfully return to my food plan. Preparation included bulking up.

Bulking up! That's the favorite pastime of professional dieters, who always start their diets on Mondays. The reason Monday is D-Day, "Diet-Day," is to enable the future dieters of America, and probably elsewhere, to have the weekend to eat all those bad foods that they have to give up while dieting. They use the weekend to fill their stomachs with chocolate bars, chips and dip, fast and fatty foods, desserts, and anything else whose calorie count per serving exceeds the maximum daily requirement.

I've bulked up many times preparing for diets, so much so that I am sure at least half my excess weight is due to this lifelong sport. I loved going on diets! It meant that prior to the deprivation I could eat all my favorite foods; I could stuff myself. And I didn't have to feel guilty!

As I embarked on this return to the program, I bulked up, but not just for a weekend. I did it for almost two whole weeks! I managed to down racks and racks of barbecued spare ribs, lots of peanut butter and jelly and margarine sandwiches, enormous steaks with French fries or baked potatoes filled with sour cream and butter, thick grilled cheese sandwiches cooked in margarine and—the *pièce de résistance* (sixteen pieces to be exact)—a butter pecan cheesecake that I hid from the rest of the family.

Although I reverted to my former bad habit of bulking up, I did make one change. I started my Food Plan for Life on a Sunday (January 9, 1994). I didn't need to wait until Monday. (Besides, I was running out of antacid tablets!)

By the way, I dubbed this get-healthy, get-fit program my Food Plan for Life because I have to follow it, with minor modifications at goal, for the rest of my life. Also, by following this healthy food plan, I will add zest to my life now and, hopefully, years to my life in the future.

SUNDAY, JANUARY 9, 1994

There's no stopping me now! I've had a little setback, but now I am ready to go forward. I have the right foods in my cupboards and refrigerator. I'm stocked up and I'm pumped up. I'm on the way and there's no turning back!

FRIDAY, JANUARY 14, 1994

I am really proud of myself. I have now gone four months without smoking. More important, I have had no desire for a cigarette in quite a while. There is another reason I feel great. I have cut down on caffeine. I used to drink an enormous number of diet colas each and every day. Some days I would go through as many as ten 12-ounce cans of diet cola. I was on a constant high, so much so that Andy, my son, would tell me I was spaced out on caffeine. Now I drink water and very few diet colas. Ever since I started drinking lots and lots of healthy water, I haven't been so jittery.

Water—H_2O. If ever there was a secret for successful weight loss, it's water. Health experts tell us that a glass of water can fill us up and flush us out. A minimum of eight glasses, 64 ounces, is the recommended daily dosage. More is even better. According to experts, if we drink lots of water before meals, we'll eat less. And, if we drink lots of water with meals, we'll eat less.

I have discovered many times when I thought I was hungry, I

was just thirsty. I reached for a large glass of water instead of food. It worked! My hunger was washed away.

SATURDAY, JANUARY 15, 1994

Went to the movies with friends, and although it was extremely tempting, I refrained from getting popcorn. This was a first. I didn't know I could enjoy a movie without eating popcorn and washing it down with a diet cola. Little successes, such as this, are helping me feel better about myself and keeping me on the road to a fit future.

FRIDAY, JANUARY 21, 1994

Good news . . . *weighed myself today. I now weigh 290 pounds. This means I'm down 20 pounds! Twelve days of complete diligence to my food plan (plus the few pounds I kept off from the fall push) have resulted in a few steps on my journey. Now I only have to lose 130 pounds!*

SUNDAY, JANUARY 23, 1994

What a fool I am! Tom and I were mad at each other for who knows what, and we didn't talk to each other all weekend. Because I was mad at Tom—and the world in general—I stuffed food into my mouth, and it wasn't healthy food. I had a peanut butter and jelly and margarine sandwich (you can see what my comfort food is). I followed this with ice cream topped with butterscotch sauce and whipped cream. Then I ate some cookies. Around 6 P.M. Tom came over and hugged me and said we were dumb to fight. (He was right!) He apologized and so did I. Tom then went to the store and bought a cherry pie (my favorite) as a peace offering. Luckily, with the fight over, I came to my senses and told him I appreciated his food gift, but I couldn't eat it because it wasn't on my food plan. He felt bad because he forgot, but then told me how proud he was of me. Since nobody else in our family likes cherry pie, Tom took it to the office the next day.

TUESDAY, JANUARY 25, 1994

Dr. Wagner reminded me how important it is to weigh and measure food. Many individuals are overweight not necessarily because of what they eat, but because they eat too much. Many times I have told others "I don't know why I'm fat. I only eat healthy foods." The problem was I ate very large portions—too large in size and calories—of these healthy foods. Measuring and weighing food can bring down my measurements and weight.

No Measuring Cup?

So you're on a deserted island, or maybe you're in a restaurant, and you don't have any measuring utensils or a food scale. No problem. Here are a few hints to help you eat the correct portion sizes.

- The size and depth of your palm is about the size of 3 ounces of cooked meats, poultry, and fish. Go to the first row of knuckles and you have an approximate 5 ounce portion.
- The tip of your finger (not your thumb) is about the size of one teaspoon.
- Cup your hand. It holds approximately 1 ounce of pretzels and almost 2 ounces of dry cereal.
- Make a fist. It's about the size of a medium fruit. Or, it's about one cup.

MONDAY, JANUARY 31, 1994

I ended the month thinking about beef. Dr. Wagner said I have to cut down on the beef and eat more seafood. I love beef—the fattier, the better. Seafood is okay, but I'm used to eating it with some kind of condiment, e.g. fish with lots of tartar sauce, lobster and crab dipped in melted butter, shrimp in lots of cocktail sauce. But that's not the way Dr. Wagner wants me to eat seafood. She wants me to eat it "naked" or with such seasonings as lemon juice or spices, things I have not yet acquired a taste for. I do eat lots of tuna fish, but I am using a small amount of regular salad dressing. Fat-free dressing, even the lite stuff, is ghastly-tasting in my opinion. I do eat more chicken than I ever did, and I will try to add more seafood to my diet. But I don't think I'll ever lose my taste for beef. As a concession, Dr. Wagner said occasionally I could have lean beef, such as round steak, but only occasionally.

During my "restart" period in January, through research I became reacquainted with the fact that eating the correct number of calories each day is instrumental to weight loss. Although I knew this from previous weight-loss ventures (that's why I have a drawer filled with books listing calorie counts), I never really understood why calories are so important.

A calorie is a measure of the amount of heat in the food we eat. It's the energy in food we use to keep our bodies working. When we eat the correct number of calories from food (and we need to factor in whether we're active or inactive), we maintain our body weight. We stay just where we are on the scale. When we consume more calories than we need, this excess energy (calories) can be stored as fat and we gain weight. Take in fewer calories than our bodies need and we lose weight.

Nutritionists once thought all calories were equal. They believed that all a person needed to do was to count calories—all calories—and if the total number was below what was needed to maintain body weight, the person would lose weight. However, new research has shown that this is not true.

Metabolically, fat calories from food rapidly convert into fats for storage, more quickly than carbohydrate and protein calories. To be successful, we need to eat a *balanced* food plan—one that limits fats. A balanced food plan with fewer calories than are needed to maintain current weight, combined with moderate exercise, will do the trick.

When I started my healthy eating program, I was fortunate to have a nutritionist who knew just how many calories I needed a day to lose weight. Based on my 300-plus pounds and the fact that I wasn't very active (something that would change), I was placed on a balanced diet of 1,800 calories a day. No wonder I lost weight. At 310 pounds, I needed 2,870 calories a day to maintain my bulk. Dr. Wagner cut these calories by 1,000, but still kept me at a healthy level. I immediately began to lose weight.

Notice the word "healthy." My new caloric intake was a "healthy" 1,800 calories. It's important that you, too, *never, ever* go below 1,200 calories a day. If you consume fewer than 1,200 calories a day, you will lose muscle tissue as well as fat. And you need muscle tissue. Muscle burns calories at twenty times the rate body fat does! Also, your body will go into a starvation mode and calories will be stored as fat. Sure, you'll lose weight at the start, but you may actually end up fatter than you were before starting your program, because the percentage of fat in your body will go up as a result of the caloric deprivation.

So how many calories of a balanced food plan do you need to

lose weight? Grab a calculator, or a pencil and paper, and using the formula below, you can determine how many calories you need at your present weight. Reducing these calories by just 500 a day can result in a weight loss of between 1 and 2 pounds a week. That's 50 pounds a year (with two weeks off for good behavior)!

How Many Calories Do You Need?

Your present weight _____
Your height (in inches) _____
Your age _____

1. Multiply your weight by 4.3. _____
2. Multiply your height (in inches) by 4.7. _____
3. Add these two numbers together plus 655. _____
4. Multiply your age by 4.7. _____
5. Subtract the number in 4 from the total in 3 _____.

This is the number of calories you need if you don't exercise. It's your resting metabolic rate, or RMR (the rate at which your body burns calories at rest). If you eat no more than this number of calories, you will not gain weight.

6. If you do moderate exercise each day—and if you want to lose weight this is a must—multiply the number of calories above by 1.4. _____ This is the total number of calories you can consume each day to maintain your present weight.

Here's how the calculation would work in the case of a forty-year-old woman who is 5 feet 4 inches tall and weighs 200 pounds.

1. $200 \times 4.3 = 860$
2. $64 \times 4.7 = 301$
3. $860 + 301 + 655 = 1,816$

4. $40 \times 4.7 = 188$
5. $1{,}816 - 188 = 1{,}628$
6. $1{,}628 \times 1.4 = 2{,}279$

If you want to lose weight at the healthy rate of at least 1 pound a week, you need to reduce your food intake by 500 calories a day. This means the woman in the example should consume no more than 1,779 calories a day for successful weight loss.

Once you've calculated the number of calories you need a day, reduce the number by 500 to lose weight. Remember . . . never go below 1,200 calories a day. If you consume fewer than 1,200 calories a day, you could slow your metabolism and sabotage your weight-loss plan.

Chapter 4

Food Plan for Life!

I'm losing weight. With a slow but sure approach (experts say weight loss is best achieved slowly, over a period of a year or more), and a food plan that is bountiful and offers lots of variety, I'm doing it. With a few minor side trips into overindulgence, I'm staying on the road.

How long was my road? How much weight did I need to lose?

When I embarked on this journey, I didn't look at those charts with suggested weights for men and women. You know, the ones that you see in diet books or hanging in doctors' offices. I didn't want anyone or anything to determine what I should weigh. I wanted to set my own goal.

When I began the *Family Circle* project, I set my goal at a weight loss of 150 pounds. Based on a 310-pound start, this goal would put me at one hundred and sixty pounds. I would then weigh about the same as my husband. (Lucky for him. I always joked with Tom that I could keep him in line by sitting on him.

Never had to, but the threat was there!) And I would be 3 pounds less than I weighed on my wedding day in 1977.

When Richard Simmons entered my life in 1996, he suggested a goal for me of 155 pounds. Based on my height, 5′7″, and my by then plus-50 age, he said this would be a healthy weight for me.

So that's what I did. I got down to 155 pounds!

After three years on my Food Plan for Life, combined with regular exercise, I realized that I could lose weight successfully. I wanted—at least once in my adult life—to be under 160 pounds. (I was in junior high school when the scale last went below that number.)

Also, never had anyone said to me that I was "too skinny." I wanted to hear these words. I wanted to feel what "too skinny" felt like.

When I chose this new goal, I did it with health in mind. I would never sacrifice good health just for a number on the scale. And at 155 pounds, I am healthy. I'm fit, healthy, and happy with this weight. I'm where I want to be!

You, too, can choose where you want to be. If you have no medical problems, you can determine your own weight-loss goal, as long as your choice is realistic and healthy. Some individuals need the guidance of a doctor or a suggested weight chart to help them in setting their goals. If you are one of these individuals, the USFDA (United States Food and Drug Administration) chart, that follows, can serve as a guide. The higher weights generally apply to men, who tend to have more muscle and bone.

USFDA Suggested Weight (without clothes or shoes)

Height	19–34 years	35 years and over
5'0"	97–128	108–138
5'1"	101–132	111–143
5'2"	104–137	115–148
5'3"	107–141	119–152
5'4"	111–146	122–157
5'5"	114–150	126–162
5'6"	118–155	130–167
5'7"	121–160	134–172
5'8"	125–164	138–178
5'9"	129–169	142–183
5'10"	132–174	146–188
5'11"	136–179	151–194
6'0"	140–184	155–199
6'1"	144–189	159–205
6'2"	148–195	164–210
6'3"	152–200	168–216
6'4"	156–205	173–222

Tuesday, February 1, 1994

My family is really important to the success of this lifestyle change. The kids have been really good about not eating junk food in front of me. More important, the family has been extremely willing (with the exception of fussy Andy) to try the low-fat meals I now make.

Friday, February 4, 1994

I lost another 2 pounds. I'm now 288 pounds. Although I feel good about this weight loss, I wish I could lose weight faster. This isn't what Dr. Wagner wants. She doesn't want me to go on a diet—she wants me to follow a healthy food plan. In the process, she promises, I will lose weight. I just wish it would go faster than it is. I want the trim body I know I have under this fat. And I want it now!

SATURDAY, FEBRUARY 12, 1994

Got off the road today; more specifically, I fell off! Went to a Chinese New Year's celebration and ate lots of egg rolls. My plan was to eat the less fattening insides of these delicacies, but I ended up eating every morsel of every one. My rationale: I didn't want to offend the hostess. (Like she even noticed!) I sure can make excuses!

SUNDAY–TUESDAY, FEBRUARY 13–15, 1994

Still off the road! My sister and I went on a three-day winter break getaway with the kids to Frankenmuth, Michigan. This town is famous for its all-you-can-eat chicken dinners and Bavarian food. Of course, I had to eat all the fattening foods. I reasoned that you don't come all the way to Frankenmuth and not eat its famous foods.

I knew I was being bad, but this guilt didn't stop me. My sister is also overweight, and she decided that this trip was her last hurrah before starting a diet. This sounded good to me. So we ate all the things we shouldn't. It's amazing how having a cohort in crime makes the crime easier. I really have to learn to be stronger. There will always be someone who wants to lead me down the fat path. Someone who wants to keep me off my road!

THURSDAY, FEBRUARY 17, 1994

With God's help and some work on my resolve, I'm back on the road to good health and fitness! I don't want to be fat anymore!

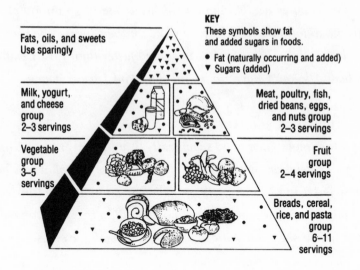

One reason I was so fat is that my favorite geometric shape for foods was the triangle. Most of my favorite foods—a piece of pizza, a piece of cheesecake, a piece of cherry pie—came in this shape. (Who am I kidding? I'd never eaten just "a piece" of pizza, cheesecake, or pie!)

Now there's a new triangle in my life. Really it's a pyramid, and it's compliments of the USDA (United States Department of Agriculture).

To me, this symbol has become an important guide to healthy eating. My 1,800-calorie food plan is based on the USDA's Food Guide Pyramid. And it should be your guide to healthy eating.

Once you've calculated the number of calories you need each day (see Chapter 3), you should make food selections based on the food pyramid. It conveys some key principles of healthy eating.

- **Eat plenty of fruits, vegetables, and grains (bread group) each day.**

- **Limit fat intake to 20–30 percent of daily calories.**
- **Cut down on meat (protein) servings.**

There's another thing you need to know to develop a healthy eating plan. You need to know how many calories are in specific foods.

It is helpful to have a book listing calories and portion sizes (percentage of fat is also important). I have one, but I don't use it very often. I find it too time-consuming looking up specific foods. Instead, I made and carry an index card containing the following information. On one side are calorie counts; on the other, serving sizes.

*Calorie Counts**

1 fat = 45 calories
1 milk = 80 calories
1 meat = 70 calories
1 vegetable = 25 calories
1 fruit = 55 calories
1 bread = 80 calories

These calorie counts are approximate.

Serving Sizes of Common Foods

1 fat = *1 teaspoon butter, margarine, mayonnaise; 1 table-spoon salad dressing, lite mayonnaise, cream cheese, whipping cream; 2 tablespoons lo-cal salad dressing, lite cream cheese, sour cream*

1 milk = *1 cup skim/nonfat milk, low-fat buttermilk, low-fat yogurt; ½ cup no-fat frozen yogurt, no-fat cottage cheese*

1 meat = *1 ounce all lean meats, poultry, fish, low-fat cheese; 1 egg; ½ cup canned (in water) tuna, salmon, or crab*

1 vegetable = *1 cup raw; ½ cup cooked*

1 fruit = *small apple, orange, peach, or pear; ½ banana, grapefruit; ⅓ cup most fruit juices*

1 bread = *1 slice regular, 2 slices diet bread; ½ bagel, English muffin, hot dog or hamburger roll; 1 small potato; ½ cup pasta, rice, cold or hot cereal*

SATURDAY, FEBRUARY 26, 1994

My Odyssey of the Mind (Libby's) team competed in the regional contest today. I knew it would be a long day, so I did what I was supposed to do. I planned. I took diet ginger ale, a couple of oranges, a tuna salad, some carrots—all the good stuff needed to stay on my food plan. My team did well, but not my diet. I ate pizza with the kids for lunch. I ate pizza with the kids for an afternoon snack. I ate pizza with the kids for dinner. I have to stop using special occasions as an excuse for going off my food plan!

Special occasions! These events are major detriments to achieving consistent weight-loss success. At least, they have been for me. Somebody's birthday, a vacation, a day trip with the kids, dinner out to celebrate this or celebrate that, lunch with a friend, a party, a wedding, a holiday, a trip to the dentist and the proclamation of "no cavities." Just about any time or any thing becomes a special occasion for me. And how do I celebrate special occasions? With food, lots and lots of food.

However, as I proceeded down my road to success, I learned how to handle special occasions better. I'm not saying I'm perfect. I'm not saying that all the obstacles have been cleared from my road, but I got to my goal (and you can get to yours) with the help of the following suggestions.

How to Successfully Handle:

PARTIES

- Plan ahead. Know that you will be tempted by the food, so eat a low-fat, low-calorie snack (vegetable soup, a vegetable salad) before you leave home.
- Drink lots of water before you leave home and when you arrive at your destination.
- Look at yourself in a mirror before you leave. Tell yourself how well you're doing and how great you look. Remind yourself that you can have a good time without eating unhealthy foods.
- Wear somewhat tight undergarments, e.g. underpants or a girdle. The small discomfort you feel will remind you of your need to be successful. (Dr. Wagner suggests wearing a belt *under* your clothes.)
- Stay away from the food table. If you don't see what you're missing, you won't miss it.
- Send your husband or a trusted friend to check the food choices. After he or she reports back to you, send him to get you healthy food.
- If it's a birthday celebration, extend best wishes with-

out eating the cake. Just say no thanks to even just one little piece.

BEING ON THE ROAD

- Always have a healthy snack (a few carrot or celery sticks, fruit, a small bag of pretzels) with you.
- Carry a fresh bottle of water in the car. Drink this instead of stopping for a soda.
- Learn the better choices you can make at fast-food restaurants (see Chapter 6).

EATING IN RESTAURANTS

- Select an establishment that serves healthy foods. (Skip places with specialties that include such fattening foods as pizza, ribs, Mexican or Chinese cuisine.)
- Plan beforehand—even before you leave for the restaurant—what you are going to eat. Make sure to follow your food plan.
- Don't even look at a menu. Stick to your planned selections.
- Tell the waitperson that, due to medical needs, you want to order "off the menu." Ask for foods cooked in broth, not oil; for broiled, not fried, meats; for steamed vegetables; for salad dressing on the side. (Never put dressing on your salad. Dip your fork into the dressing first, then pick up a bite of salad.)
- Skip the roll and butter.
- Drink lots of water before and during the meal.

- When your meal arrives, ask for a carryout container. Immediately, before you begin eating, place the extra amount of food (if the portion size is too large, and it usually is) in the container to take home.
- Don't order dessert. (It's usually too expensive anyway!)

HOLIDAYS

- If you're the host/hostess, plan the meal to include some healthy food offerings.
- Send leftover desserts and other high-calorie, high-fat foods home with your guests.
- If you're a guest, check with the host/hostess about the menu. Offer to bring some healthy food choices. (Also, bring some good foods for the appetizer course.)
- Drink lots of water before and during the meal.

VACATIONS

- As part of your travel plans, *plan* to not take a vacation from healthy eating.
- Ask the locals where you can get healthy foods.
- Enjoy where you are, not what you're eating!
- Drink lots of water. If necessary, take bottled water with you.

SUNDAY, MARCH 13, 1994

I have discovered a secret to success. When I first started the food plan, I would find a food, such as broccoli slaw, that I really liked and I would eat it all the time. Now I know that variety is important. I used to eat broccoli slaw as much as five times a day. I did the same thing with baked apples and baked potatoes with vegetables, no-fat refried beans and salsa. I'd find a food I liked, then I would eat it time and time again. I reached the point where I could hardly look at broccoli slaw, baked apples, baked potatoes, and a number of other things. Now I've learned that variety helps give me a healthy interest in food, the right foods. I now vary the cereals I eat each morning, the fruits, the vegetables, and the meats. I don't eat the same things day in and day out. I'm even trying new things, things I didn't think I would like. Some I do; some I don't.

WEDNESDAY, MARCH 16, 1994

This program is working in a number of positive ways. My choles-terol was almost 250 when I began the program in September. Now my level is 175 with an LDL/HDL ratio of 4.5 (female average range is 3.7–5.6). Dr. Wagner said at the rate I'm going, I will live to one hundred years of age!

FRIDAY, APRIL 1, 1994

The day to weigh! I try to weigh only on the first day of of every month. I've lost another 2 pounds. I've hit the magic 30! I've lost 30 pounds, and I feel better than I did when I was thirty years of age. I walk now like a young woman. I have bounce in my step.

For the past ten years I've walked "old." I've waddled. Because of this, friends and strangers tended to treat me as if I were old and handicapped. They rushed to open doors. They extended arms for support. They walked slower so I wouldn't be left behind. Now I

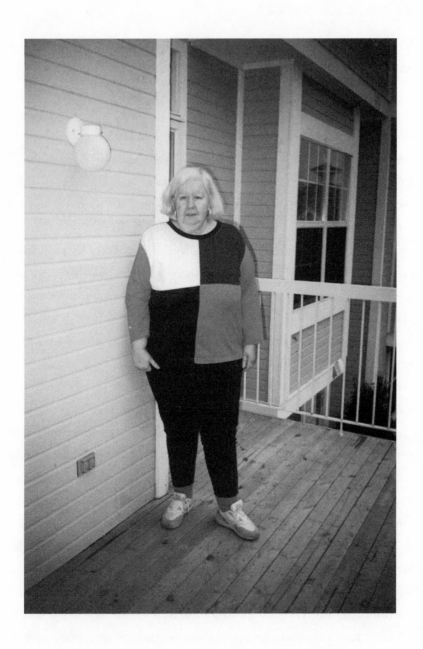

Down 28 pounds in the spring of 1994. I'm not happy because it's going so slowly.

have a little hop and bop to my step. Some of it comes from the 30-pound weight loss; much comes from knowing that I am succeeding.

THURSDAY, APRIL 7, 1994

I'm depressed. Again, I feel this program—this journey—should be going faster. I feel that losing 30 pounds isn't enough. I know that if I were on a diet I would have lost a lot more weight. I shared these thoughts with Dr. Wagner. She reminded me of the reason why I am losing weight slowly. "Fast" pounds come back fast.

I was proud to tell Dr. Wagner that I passed up cheesecake, a favorite, on Easter. She said that success comes "not only by not eating cheesecake, but also by reaching the point of not wanting it." Will I ever reach that point?

Dr. Wagner reinforced the reason for my high-calorie food plan versus a low-calorie diet. She said the 1,800-calorie food plan will bring success. The amount of food I am able to eat allows me to feel satisfied and thereby decreases the chance for failure.

Also, unlike some diets that allow you to eat a certain amount of proteins, fruits, breads, etc. a day, this food plan provides certain foods for each meal and each snack. For breakfast I am allowed two bread servings in the form of cold cereal. I cannot save these bread servings for later in the day. If I don't eat them for breakfast (which is a no-no), I don't get them later. They're lost. I can only eat for breakfast, lunch, and dinner what is specified for each of these meals. Even if I am going to a party later at night, I cannot save anything. At the party, I am only allowed to eat my night snack, which is two bread servings, and some vegetables, which are unlimited.

The food plan I was following is not unique. Like all healthy and balanced food plans designed to aid weight loss, it is based on a safe caloric intake, snacks for those times when food cravings are at their peak, a variety of foods and portions that enabled me to feel satisfied and full. My food plan consisted of:

BREAKFAST
1 fruit
2 bread servings
1 milk

MORNING SNACK
1 bread serving

LUNCH
4 ounces of meat
1-plus vegetables
2 bread servings
1 fruit
1 fat serving

AFTERNOON SNACK
2 bread servings

DINNER
6 ounces of meat
1-plus vegetables
2 bread servings
1 fruit
1 fat serving
1 milk

EVENING SNACK
2 bread servings

This food plan may be for you. (But check with your doctor first!) It allows you to choose your foods. If you're like me, being able to choose foods you like will help you stay on the program. You'll make it down the road to success.

Chapter 5

Getting a Leg Up
with Exercise!

Following my food plan was leading to success, but it wasn't the only reason. Activation (in the form of exercise) was leading to realization. Exercise was moving me down the road to my goal. And no wonder. The combination of aerobic and resistance exercises and a lower-calorie food plan results in increased energy expenditure, increased fat burning, and decreased fat storage. This means you lose weight faster and better.

I started slowly, very, very slowly, by walking first one mile, then two, around the neighborhood. In the beginning, it took me half an hour or more to complete one mile. A slug, after all, isn't known for its speed!

Then a wonderful thing happened. A local club—Beverly Hills Racquet and Health Club—offered me and my family a free membership. As part of its community service mission, it wanted to help me. In addition, I would have a trainer to set up and oversee an appropriate fitness program. This slug was going to have a personal trainer, at least to get me started! The thought was almost unthinkable, even laughable.

Although somewhat nervous about the prospect of working out in a spandex, thong environment with slim, trim, and muscular fitness addicts, I was also excited. I could visualize my body getting not only smaller but also firmer. "Firm." Now there's a word that had never been used to describe my body!

The first few weeks at the health club were hard. I thought everybody was staring at me and thinking, "What is that fat lady doing here?" However, as difficult as it was, both physically and emotionally, I went at least four times a week. I did what I was told by the trainer. I wanted this to work.

I had another problem with working out at the health club. What does a fat lady wear? Luckily, a trip to a popular retail store provided the answer. I found inexpensive pants and tops in plus sizes that would cover my 300-pound body. The T-shirt tops were large and long enough to handle my expansive bottom. The pants worked, too. And these coverings came in lots of bright colors. (Forget those dark "fat-hiding" colors; I wanted to look cheerful and optimistic.) I bought four outfits, one for each day I worked out. These, and some additions in even brighter colors, would be my uniform for the next four years.

I had the place to go, the clothes to wear, a trainer. And I had the determination. I was ready!

MONDAY, APRIL 18, 1994

Another 2 pounds have come off! (I sneaked on the scale!) Now I'm 32 pounds lighter. Working out and following a good food plan is truly the answer. I'm a believer.

Some friends have said I'm losing weight because I have all this help—a nutritionist and trainers. I do agree that these people are helpful, but I'm doing the real work. I'm the one who decides what goes into my mouth. Nobody prepares my meals. I'm the one who pushes myself to the health club to work out. I'm doing the sweating and I'm choosing to eat healthy foods.

SATURDAY, APRIL 30, 1994

The month is ending on a great note. Food choices are excellent. Exercise is becoming almost enjoyable. At least I feel good after I exercise, except for my feet. They hurt. My children and husband are extremely proud of me, especially my husband. He's been more snuggly and he pinches my fanny on a regular basis. (He never did that before!)

My daughter Emily said she's happy I'm going to be a "regular" mom, because some of the kids have said I was fat. She said she never told me this before because she didn't want to hurt me. "But," she said, "I can tell you now, because you're getting skinny."

I needed to buy a new outfit this week and I fit into a size 22. That's size 22 in both slacks and top. This is a nice change from my former 26s and 28s!

When I first began to exercise at the club, the trainer put me on the treadmill. He said walking was enough. I tried walking for five minutes at a very slow speed. I made it, but just barely. Each time I went to the club, the trainer added a few more minutes, until I could walk comfortably for fifteen minutes. Once I got comfortable, the time and speed were increased. Slow but sure. I was becoming physically fit.

To provide for all my fitness needs, the trainer soon added

weight training as well as basic aerobic classes, including water aerobics. I was beginning to feel like a jock, a very healthy jock.

Walking on the treadmill might be healthy, but it also was taking a toll on me. I developed my first ever sports injury—tendonitis in my heels. Although in tremendous pain, I didn't stop walking. (My trainer bandaged my feet to help alleviate the pain.) I was committed. I didn't want the pain to interfere with the great strides I was making.

Fitting fitness into a very hectic schedule, especially with a husband and three active kids, was not easy. However, with a little juggling and family cooperation, it didn't take long to make it a habit. Behavioral experts have found it takes approximately twenty-one days for a fitness commitment to "take." And, if you exercise at least three or four days a week, at the same time each day, for three weeks in a row, you're more apt to stay with it for the long term.

Even if you, like me, are on a tight schedule, you should be able to find time for a few ten-minute workout segments each day. Add up those ten-minute segments and you can easily meet the thirty minutes a day necessary for fitness.

If you work outside the home, turn your coffee break into an exercise break. Walk up and down the stairs or outside for ten minutes. If neither of these options is available, go into the rest room and march in place. Take your exercise shoes out for lunch. Walk or jog for ten or twenty minutes.

A few minutes of movement here and there add up to a more active lifestyle. Be creative and activate your daily routines by using the stairs when possible, parking your car at the far end of the parking lot, delivering inner-office messages in person instead of using the telephone or e-mail.

You have lots of exercising options at home. Pop an aerobic

tape into your VCR and follow along, even if you can only do a few minutes at a time. Invite a neighbor or friend to go for a walk. Get a rope and jump for at least five minutes each day. Turn on the radio and dance. Doing the twist provides a good aerobic exercise at the same time it works on your waist. (Hold your tummy in and you'll have even better results!) March in place in front of the television during your favorite show. Or use commercial breaks as exercise time. Get up and do some jumping jacks (you know, those things we had to do long ago in gym class).

I have found an excellent way to stay active. I have discovered books on tape, especially mysteries. I allow myself to listen to these books only when I am exercising. Once I get into a book, especially a mystery, I find I exercise longer. I lose myself in the book instead of looking at the clock to see if I'm just about done. Others have found listening to music to be just as effective.

Commit to Get Fit

- *Make exercise a priority.* Think of physical activity as an essential body upkeep like brushing your teeth, showering, fixing your hair.
- *Find the time.* Look at your daily schedule. With some rearranging, you should be able to discover at least thirty minutes each day for exercise. If need be, cut down on nonessential telephone calls or just one half-hour television show.
- *Select a specific time.* Whether it's in the morning or later in the day, choose the same time each day to exercise. This way exercise becomes a regular daily habit. (Experts say individuals who work out in the mornings are more apt to stick with their programs than those who

leave it to later. Unplanned obstacles often eliminate "later.")

- ***Wear the proper shoes and clothes.*** Get good shoes (see an expert for help) and wear comfortable clothes.
- ***Don't procrastinate!*** Get rid of excuses. There's no reason not to do something good for yourself by making exercise one of your daily priorities. Set exercise goals—small and reasonable ones at first—and then work to achieve them.

MONDAY, MAY 2, 1994

Taped another Maury Povich Show. The show's guests included two overweight women who wanted to meet me. They had written to Family Circle *after my weight-loss journey was announced in the January issue. These women told me I was their inspiration and they asked for my assistance. I realized what a responsibility I have to others. I'm very excited about my success (I've now lost 35 pounds, based on the* Family Circle *start of 310, and 50 pounds, based on my highest weight of 325 pounds at the start of 1993), and I feel like a preacher who wants to share the good news with everyone. However, I know I can't help anyone unless they want to help themselves. They have to be motivated and willing to do what it takes to achieve success. I wish I had been motivated when I was in my thirties or even my early forties, but I wasn't. That's why the diets didn't work. It took reaching almost fifty years of age to realize that my excess weight was affecting my health. This is what motivated me.*

FRIDAY, MAY 27, 1994

Ring the bells! Beat the drums! Today marks a major achievement! I was visiting with my daughter's principal today and without realizing it, I crossed my legs. I crossed my legs! I haven't been able to do that in years. Ain't life grand when you live right!

MEMORIAL DAY WEEKEND, MAY 28–30, 1994

I realized something wonderful. The age of fifty is not an old-age sentence. These days fifty is the prime of life. This age means a person, with luck and health, has a third of his or her life to go. Imagine, having the wisdom that comes with fifty years and still having twenty-five, thirty, or even forty or more years to go. This is why it's so important to be healthy and fit at fifty. I want to spend all the rest of my years with a minimum of old-age pain and with enough energy to do the things I want to do.

On Memorial Day I was in charge of two floats for our village parade. I decided to walk the parade route (almost two miles) next to one of the floats. I knew I could do it. All that exercise was paying off. Many friends and neighbors noticed me in the parade and offered wonderful praise and words of encouragement. For almost the whole distance I walked on air, even though my tendonitis was killing me. I felt like the most svelte woman there. Then, reality hit. Toward the end of the parade, a small boy burst my bubble. "Mom, look at that fat lady," he said, pointing to me. At first I was hurt. Then I realized I needed that comment. Although I have made progress, I still have a distance to go . . . I still have a long journey on the road to my goal. But I'll get there! Yes, little boy, the fat lady will reach the end of the road and she'll be more fit.

WEDNESDAY, JUNE 1—SUNDAY, JUNE 5, 1994

On the road to Iowa State University for Odyssey of the Mind world finals. I'm on the state board for this program that challenges students to solve engineering and creative problems. I am really proud of myself. The whole trip included eating in fast-food restaurants and

I succeeded in eating well and right! The only upsetting thing about the trip was that I couldn't exercise on a regular basis. I was in the car too much. I can't believe I miss my exercise routine.

MONDAY, JUNE 6, 1994

I'm back to exercise. Thank heaven! And I reached another "low point" today. I have now lost 40 pounds! More important, I am still motivated. Also, I made the cover of Family Circle. *Imagine. A cover girl!*

SUNDAY, JUNE 12, 1994

Celebrated Andy's fifteenth birthday with a family (twenty-two people) dinner. My mother, who has always been fixated on my weight and heavy people in general (she's super slim and eats healthy and at seventy-one years of age exercises daily), said she can't believe how I now move around. "You hardly sit down anymore," she said. She reminded me that in the past when I entertained, everybody else did the work. People waited on me and treated me as if I were handicapped. Now I'm up and moving (thanks a little to the weight loss and a lot to the exercise). I'm not sure if this is an advantage. Everyone left without helping me clean up!

MONDAY, JUNE 27, 1994

I am so proud of myself. My right foot continues to throb with pain, but I continue to exercise. (My doctor gave me some exercises to help the tendonitis and they're doing some good. Also, binding my foot before I exercise lessens the pain.) I like how I feel after I finish working out. I feel alive!

I got on the scale today. I couldn't wait until the first! Now it's 45 pounds that I've lost! How exciting! I haven't been this low since . . . , heaven knows when!

TUESDAY, JULY 5, 1994

Today I did my usual half-hour walk (at 2.7 miles per hour) with the treadmill elevated to 5. When I finished, my body didn't feel as "worked" as it normally does. Then I noticed I had forgotten to set the elevation. I did an amazing thing—amazing for me, anyway. I got right back on the treadmill, made the correct settings, and walked another half hour. Where oh where has the slug gone?

I can't believe how exercise has become such an important part of my life in such a short period of time. I can't believe that I go to the health club, or high school track, at least five times a week, and sometimes seven days, to sweat. (I used to sweat before, but that was because of the excess weight I was carrying around. I am still over-weight—I am, after all, 265 pounds—but I sweat now because I work out. And this sweat is "sweeter!")

Exercise has definitely improved my quality of life. That's a major benefit of exercise. But it's not the only one.

The Benefits of Exercise

- Reduces the risk of dying prematurely.
- Reduces the risk of heart disease.
- Reduces the risk of developing diabetes.
- Reduces the risk of developing high blood pressure.
- Helps reduce blood pressure for those with high blood pressure.
- Reduces the risk of developing colon cancer.
- Reduces the risk of developing breast cancer.
- Improves immune system functioning.
- Reduces abdominal obesity.
- Helps build and maintain healthy bones, muscles, and joints.

- Helps control weight.
- Burns excess calories.
- Increases muscle endurance.
- Improves balance and coordination.
- Prevents constipation.
- Improves posture.
- Helps alleviate back pain.
- Improves sleep.
- Slows signs of aging.
- Helps older adults become stronger and more agile.
- Reduces feelings of depression, stress, and anxiety.
- Promotes psychological well-being.
- Improves mental sharpness.
- Increases energy, stamina, and vigor.

According to *A Report of the Surgeon General on Physical Activity and Health* (1996), individuals who are usually inactive can improve their health and well-being by becoming even moderately active on a regular basis. Also, physical activity need not be strenuous to achieve health benefits. For those who already participate in some exercise, greater health benefits can be achieved by increasing the frequency, duration, or intensity of physical activity.

I no longer need the Surgeon General or other health experts to tell me that exercise is good for me. I know this firsthand. I learned it soon after I began regular participation in an exercise program. Exercise makes me and my body feel good!

The value of exercise has become apparent in my everyday life. It's no longer difficult to get in and out of the bathtub, to shave my legs, to tie my shoes, to pick up dropped objects, to carry groceries, to put up wallpaper, to clean above, below, and behind things, to get in and out of cars (especially backseats), or to do a million other tasks that were impossible before my involvement in physical activity.

Exercise means everything when it comes to doing just about anything. If you learn this, as I have, and you get active, you, too, can begin to live a full life, a new and improved life. Exercise makes all the difference!

Chapter 6

Just Doing It!

I was doing everything I needed to do to reach my goal. I was following the food plan; I was exercising. And I was losing weight and getting healthy in the process. However, I can't say I was having fun. This wasn't a walk in the park.

Losing weight is hard work. Eating healthy on a consistent basis and exercising every day take determination. I was in constant fear that I would give up, I would fail. There were just too many challenges, too many obstacles. I hadn't been successful in the past. What made me think I would reach my goal this time?

In addition to the fear of failure for myself, I worried about the *Family Circle* readers and the television viewers who were counting on me. I knew, especially from the hundreds of letters I received, that many overweight women were looking to me as a guide to their own success. If I succeeded, they believed they, too, could succeed. If I failed, my failure would be their excuse for failure. After all, if I didn't make it with all this help, how could they be expected to achieve their goals?

The pressure at times took its toll. I reverted to the bad habits of a lifetime—I turned to bingeing to handle the stress. Then I spent hours immersed in guilt. So then I overate again . . . then, again, the guilt.

Luckily, I didn't gain weight. I never gave up the exercise. It had become such an important part of my life that, no matter what happened with the food, I continued to work out on a regular basis. As a result, I maintained my weight.

However, staying at the same weight would never get me to my goal. It was time to move beyond the pressure and to move down the scale. It was time for a new tactic, something that would work.

Visualization had worked in the past. It could and would work again. I needed a new picture to focus on, a new mental image.

I knew I had to grit my teeth if I were to move farther down the road. That's it! I created a mental picture of myself holding my teeth tightly together with a renewed determination. If my teeth were clenched, unhealthy food would not be able to get into my mouth. I visualized only healthy food passing my lips. Whenever I was tempted to binge or overindulge, I saw my clenched teeth. It worked, and still does when my resolve weakens.

I envision myself gritting my teeth at those times, such as eating out, when being good is extremely hard.

One of the greatest challenges of weight loss is eating out, especially in restaurants. Although I have discovered ways of making this less difficult (see Chapter 4), I wish I had a card to hand to waitpersons and other food providers that proclaims:

In case you haven't noticed, I am an overweight person.
Please do not serve me any high-calorie or high-fat foods.
Thank you for your assistance.

I don't carry such a card, so I must make my own decisions about food. And I'm getting better with my choices. I'm learning that eating out doesn't mean my food plan is out!

MONDAY, JULY 18, 1994

Tom wants to make vacation plans, but I'm holding back. I don't feel secure yet about making food decisions while I'm on vacation. I still use the word "vacation" to mean a getaway from a healthy lifestyle.

I have to learn that I need to follow my food plan each and every day of my life—that there are no exceptions. I have to learn that the word "vacation" stands for a "different routine," but one that includes healthy food.

Tom is great. He understood my reluctance and told me we'll go on vacation when I am ready. "No big deal," he said.

Another reason I dread vacations is that all our vacations have included numerous stops at fast-food restaurants. I just don't do well at these eateries.

I'd like to say that, in the interest of health, the Prysbys have given up all fast-food restaurants. But I don't think that will ever happen. Fast foods fit into our busy schedules and, at times, are a necessity. There are some situations when I am sure we wouldn't eat if there wasn't a fast-food place to drive through or run into. Besides, who ever heard of a kid existing without an occasional burger, fries, or taco?

We still make fast-food runs, but now we make healthier food choices, especially me. I've learned what I can eat (basically salads with light vinaigrette dressings, chicken sandwiches without dressing, and an occasional chicken soft taco or baked potato with a small-size chili on top), and I know what to avoid ("super" burgers, especially with cheese and sauce, pizza, and those ever popular fries). Below are the food choices I make at the fast-food restaurants I patronize.

My Fast-Food Choices

CHOICE	CALORIES	FAT GRAMS
McDonald's •		
Garden Salad	35	0.0
with Fat-Free Herb or	0	0.0
Lite Vinaigrette Dressing	50	2.0
Grilled Chicken Salad	120	1.5
with Lite Vinaigrette Dressing	50	2.0
Hamburger on Roll	260	9.0
Grilled Chicken Deluxe Sandwich		
(Plain)	300	5.0
Burger King •		
BK Broiler Chicken Sandwich Without		
Sauce	250	8.0
Garden Salad	90	0.0
with Reduced-Calorie		
Italian Dressing	15	0.5
Hamburger on Roll	310	12.0
Wendy's •		
Baked Potato (Plain)	310	0.0
with Small Chili	210	7.0
Junior Hamburger on Roll	270	10.0
Grilled Chicken Salad	200	8.0

Deluxe Garden Salad	110	6.0
with Fat-Free French Dressing	35	0.0
with Reduced-Calorie, Reduced-Fat		
Italian Dressing	40	3.0
Grilled Chicken Breast Sandwich	310	8.0

Taco Bell •

Chicken Soft Taco	250	11.0
Light Chicken Soft Taco	180	5.0
Regular Taco	170	10.0
Regular Soft Taco	210	10.0

Kentucky Fried Chicken •

Tender Roast Breast and Drumstick		
(skin removed)	236	6.7
Small Coleslaw	180	9.0
Mashed Potatoes and Gravy	120	6.0
Garden Rice	75	1.0

Arby's •

Roasted Chicken Deluxe Sandwich	276	6.0
Roast Beef Deluxe Sandwich	296	10.0

Pizza (an average from various restaurants)

2 Slices Cheese Pizza		
from Large (16″) Pie	400	12.0

Subway •
6-inch Sandwiches on Wheat Bread:

Turkey	290	4.0
Ham	300	5.0
Club (cold cuts)	315	5.0
Roast Beef	315	5.0
Salads:		
Vegetable	55	1.0
Turkey	100	2.0
Club (with cold cuts)	125	3.0

> NOTE: *The calorie and fat counts are estimates. If you have specific medical problems, such as hypertension, food choices should be based not only on calories and fat content, but also on sodium levels. (Fast foods are known for their high salt content.) Check the nutritional guides provided by the restaurants.*

I don't like to eat breakfast out, especially at fast-food restaurants. There aren't very many healthy choices for this first meal of the day, and I don't like spending money on cereal. Formerly, when I ate breakfast out, I tended to bypass the cereal and opt for fattening fried eggs, hash browns, and bacon, sausage, or ham (or all three, if they were offered on the special). And no matter how strong my resolve, I ordered those egg, cheese, and sausage breakfast sandwiches. The ones loaded with fats and calories.

Now, if I am in a situation where I have to eat breakfast out, I choose either a small (½ cup) orange juice (56 calories; 0.2 fat grams) or an 8-ounce (1 cup) skim milk (86 calories; 0.4 fat grams). With these beverages, I select one of the following:

A plain bagel—it counts as two breads—(160 calories; 1.5 fat grams), or

An English muffin—it counts as two breads—(180 calories; 3.6 fat
  grams), or
Two slices of toast (160 calories; 2.2 fat grams).

On these breads I use one tablespoon of margarine (100 calories; 11 fat grams) or, if available, light or diet margarine with half
the calories (50) and half the fat grams (5.5). I also use one table-
spoon of jam or jelly (50 calories and no fat grams).

Planning (there's that word again) what I eat, even if my
choices are from fast-food establishments, has enabled me to lose
weight. With the weight loss have come some major and minor
changes, all of which are good.

WEDNESDAY, JULY 20, 1994

*I am going to get real personal today. One of the best things about
losing weight has to do with my personal hygiene. When I got to 300
pounds, I found that I had urine leakage on a regular basis, so much
so that I had to wear feminine napkins. I could not admit that I was
incontinent. That only happens to older individuals. I never men-
tioned this problem to my doctor. I was too embarrassed.*

*But I can mention it now, because it's gone. With the loss of 45
pounds has come an end to the leakage. Now I know I was not
incontinent. It was the excess weight. I am sure the exercise has also
helped. Whatever . . . I feel great freedom!*

SATURDAY, JULY 30, 1994

A few other things have come with the weight loss.

*Without even realizing it, I no longer drive around parking lots
waiting for one of the close spots to become available. I now drive
into lots and take whatever spot is available, whether it's up front or
in the back. I have the ability to walk now without getting winded.*

Also, I now wear blouses with button closures down the front. I haven't been able to wear a button-down blouse in years. When I tried to wear this kind of top, I needed to "safety pin" the gaping spaces between the buttonholes, or—and this happened a few times—the material pulled so badly at the buttonholes that it ripped. Definitely not a pretty sight! The other day I put on a new blouse (size 22, thank you!) and it buttoned very easily. More important, the blouse lay flat with no pulling down the front, no gaps, no nothing. It was great to look down the front of me and see that it lay flat, and that the blouse wasn't tight. I felt small in it.

The toll of excess weight extends in all directions—personal hygiene, walking even short distances, clothes. These and a score of other things have been impacted by my excess weight. Some of the most mundane, but necessary, tasks of everyday life become almost insurmountable when you're obese.

For years, no matter how high the temperature, I wore long pants and tops with sleeves. True, my body size was hardly fit for shorts and sleeveless tops, but that wasn't the only reason for the coverage. The other was body hair. It was just too difficult to shave my legs, and my arms hurt to hold them up to shave under my arms. It was just easier to cover up.

Also, and this is really embarrassing, keeping myself clean was difficult. The excessive weight made it almost impossible to reach certain areas of my body. I did the best I could, and I relied on showers to do the job. However, I spent many days worrying and hoping that I didn't smell. And I used a lot of deodorant and perfumes. What an awful way to live!

Monday, August 1, 1994

I weighed myself today. Boy! Am I depressed. I haven't lost any more weight. I know I've done so well, yet it's still only 45 pounds. Maybe, without telling Dr. Wagner, I should cut my calories down to 900 or 1,000 a day. Then I'll really lose weight. My fiftieth birthday is in November and I want to at least reach the halfway mark of 75 pounds.

Thursday, August 4, 1994

Thank heavens I didn't do anything stupid, like cutting back on my calories. I met with Dr. Wagner today and she set me straight. I have reached that well-known dieter's obstacle—the dreaded plateau. But, and Dr. Wagner stressed the importance of this, never, ever reduce calories. Doing this is how dieters fail. They reduce their calories, then they become hungry, then they overeat, then success becomes unattainable.

Dr. Wagner assured me that the plateau was only temporary and I will begin losing weight again. She said that I was probably at 265 pounds for some period in my life and the body "remembers" this, so that's the reason I've stopped losing. To assist me with further weight loss, she again stressed that I must weigh and measure my food portions to make sure I am following the food plan properly. Also, she said I must write down everything I am going to eat and plan my food consumption the night before. She reduced my dinner meat portion from six to four ounces. This, she said, should help.

Saturday, August 6, 1994

Stopped at a doughnut shop today with Libby. I had one of those coupons that gave you six free if you buy six. I just love saving money! So I bought a dozen. Libby ate one, that's all she wanted. I ate six of them before I had traveled the four miles back to my house. If that wasn't bad enough, when I got home I felt so guilty that I went to the bathroom and made myself throw up. Then I was really afraid. I have never done this before. It was something I didn't want to do, but I kept thinking that the doughnuts were going to increase my weight.

I've been depressed because I am on a plateau and now, thanks to my weakness, I am probably going to gain weight. That's why I made myself throw up.

Over the years I have made jokes about my weight. I do this so that people won't laugh at me but will laugh with me instead. So I was always the first to tell fat jokes. One of my jokes—I made it up myself—was to tell people I was bulimic. Then when my audience looked at me in astonishment, I would say, "I just don't purge!" I got the laughs with that one. But today I purged. How low can I get?

Making ourselves the butt (now there's a nice word) of fat jokes is one way we handle our obesity. If we bring up our weight first and say something funny, then, maybe, we don't have to worry about possible attacks from others. If family and friends think we are comfortable with being overweight, so comfortable, in fact, that we can joke about it, then our weight must not be a problem. Besides, fat people are supposed to be jovial!

Everyone knows that fat people are funny, and everyone wants to be around happy, funny individuals. It's our duty to carry on this stereotype. And I've done my share.

But most overweight people are not happy with themselves. There are a few who go on talk shows and tell the television world that being fat is wonderful and that they are happy with their size and themselves. But whom are they kidding?

I was one of those who portrayed herself as a happy and funny person. I was one of those jovial individuals whom everyone wanted to be around . . . I was fun. However, I was *never* happy with my weight. I *never* thought it was funny to be so large that little kids and adults alike stared at me when I entered a room or walked down the street.

My excess weight has always made me sad. I just didn't show this side of myself to others. Why wreck the image! Maybe people wouldn't like me if I wasn't funny and always so happy. So, the jokes about "this fat lady"—me—kept coming.

THURSDAY, AUGUST 11, 1994

This plateau is driving me crazy. I weigh myself every day (a no-no, according to Dr. Wagner) and the scale just doesn't move. Not upward; not downward!

I asked my trainer if I should increase my exercise and try to burn up more calories. He said to continue what I'm doing, no more. And, according to him, what I am doing is the right way to get healthy and to reduce my weight. If more exercise were added, he said, I would soon tire of it and it would no longer be fun. Then I might give up exercise totally.

SATURDAY, AUGUST 13, 1994

My son, Andy, returned from football camp today. I discovered that he had taken an issue of Family Circle *magazine with him to camp. (I'll bet this is the first teenage boy who has ever taken a women's magazine to football camp.) This particular issue had my picture and progress in it. Andy said he was so proud of what I am doing that he took it to show his friends. What a kid!*

FRIDAY, AUGUST 19, 1994

I now look forward to breakfast each and every morning. I never ate breakfast before. Even as a little kid it was my least favorite meal. I didn't like the full and uncomfortable feeling that food gave me first thing in the morning. Now I eat breakfast every day. It gives me the get-up-and-go that has been touted for years. It also keeps my system operating like clockwork.

Another amazing thing is that my taste buds have adjusted so well to less fat in my diet that I do not like some of my former favorite foods. Two percent milk now tastes too rich and too creamy. I much prefer ¹/₂ percent or skim milk. Also, I can't handle the taste of French fries. I sneaked a few of the kids', but they tasted yucky.

This food plan has done another thing for me. It has turned me into a cook, and a creative one at that. Prior to the food plan, our family meals were quite standard—meat (lots), potatoes (lots), salad and/or vegetables (small amount), and dessert. Now I actually make good dishes. Dishes that are more nutritious. Dishes the family likes. Also, I have added a number of vegetables and fruits to our diet— some that we've never used before. Zucchini and summer squash are frequent additions to stir-fry dishes and salads.

The family as a whole is receiving the benefits of my lifestyle change. They have a more active wife and mother, healthier meals, and a cleaner house (because I now have more energy). In my previous life, I joked that I kept my house "just above code so they wouldn't take the kids away." (I added, on those days when the kids were particularly troublesome, I would go "below code" and then make an anonymous call to social services. But they never came to take the kids away!)

My housekeeping methods, although not as bad as some, had not been very good. I just hadn't had the strength to keep the house picture-perfect. My excess weight got in the way of scrubbing floors, washing windows, and other more difficult household chores. I did the best I could, and my husband filled in whenever possible. (How lucky for me that I married a fit and willing husband!)

MONDAY, AUGUST 22–FRIDAY, AUGUST 26, 1994

This was a week of discoveries. Although I am still on a plateau (I think! I refuse to weigh myself anymore!), I am enjoying the changes in my body. When I look down at my feet I can now see my toes. I no longer see my stomach sticking out.

Speaking of my stomach . . . When I was younger I was overweight. About the only time I felt skinny was when I was lying in bed. Then my stomach would go flat. (Maybe I just had a droopy mattress and my rear sank down into it!) I would feel really glamorous lying in bed as a teenager. I only wished back then that I had long, silky hair to spread out on the pillow. I haven't been able to have this feeling as an adult. My stomach got so big that even when I lay down on my bed, it would be a big round ball. In fact, sitting, standing, or lying down, my stomach was so large I looked pregnant all the time.

Now my stomach is flat. I might still be big, but my stomach is flat! I have captured that glamorous feeling of my youth when I lie down on the bed. Because of this, I have felt more appealing to my husband. We are enjoying each other again. I can hardly wait until I've lost another 100 pounds. We're going to have to sleep in separate beds or we won't get any sleep!

Another discovery. I have to iron my knit outfits. I, like a number of other heavy individuals, wear knits because they stretch to fit whatever size we are. For a number of years, I haven't had to worry about ironing these knits. I was so big, my body stretched out all the wrinkles. Not anymore! The knit outfits are loose on me, so the wrinkles show. I'm back to the ironing board!

One more thing. My car has a knob by the floor on the driver's side that can be pressed to release the hatch covering the gas tank. I could never reach this knob without opening the car door. My hips were just too big. Now I don't have to open the door. I can reach it easily!

WEDNESDAY, AUGUST 31, 1994

I am ending this month no longer depressed because I am still on this plateau. I am doing what I should be doing and that's all I can ask of myself. I called up a mental picture to take off the pressure of being on the plateau.

I visualize myself on a mountain range, a beautiful place. I have climbed to the top of one of the tallest mountains (this represents my great mass of fat) and now I am climbing down. If I come down too fast there is the chance that I'll hurt myself. So I descend slowly. I have been climbing down and now, through no fault of my own, I have reached a plateau and I have been here for a long period of time. At first, in my mental picture and in reality, I was angry and depressed, pacing back and forth on the plateau and not getting anywhere. Then I saw myself sitting down and enjoying the view. I may not be getting anywhere right at this moment, but I am building up my reserves, both physically and spiritually, for the rest of the journey down the mountain.

This mental picture has relieved the stress. It has also allowed me the opportunity to appreciate my success and to reinforce my resolve for future success.

THURSDAY, SEPTEMBER 1, 1994

I celebrated an important anniversary today. One year of not smoking. *Who said you can't give up smoking and lose weight at the same time? I feel great about this success, but as much as I would like to* say that I don't miss cigarettes, I still do. I love how I feel without them. I love how clear my voice is now. I love the fact that I don't cough in the morning and many times throughout the day. I love all this, but I still miss smoking. I will not, *however*, start this revolting habit again. *I'm done for life!*

Chapter 7

From Woes to WOWS!

What a difference a year makes!

Just twelve months ago I weighed more than 300 pounds and I was desperate. I feared I was on the path to poor health and, possibly, even a premature death. I was not only tired of dragging around so much weight, it was pulling me down both physically and emotionally. That's when I turned to *Family Circle*. I needed help, and the magazine came through.

Now it was my turn to help. I was given the wonderful opportunity to guide other overweight women down the road to success.

TUESDAY, SEPTEMBER 6, 1994

I can hardly believe it. I asked the health club if I could form an exercise class for overweight women. The club eagerly agreed. I would be the inspiration and the motivation. A trainer would handle the perspiration. The class would be named after me and be called WOWS (Work Out With Sandra). I added the slogan "It's only fitting!"

If anyone had told me I would ever lead an exercise class, I would have told them they were nuts. The slug leading an exercise class! Never! However, now this slug has turned fitness expert, and I have the opportunity to help other women by sharing my secrets for success. Helping others has always been my nature, so this is perfect. Besides, the classes will give me new incentive for staying on track.

Exercise classes specifically geared for overweight women are truly needed, but rare. I know this because I never found one that focused on my needs—one that took into account my extreme excess weight.

Once, when I was about 225 pounds, I tried a "lite" aerobic class. It was billed as an "easy, fun way to exercise for the beginner." What I discovered in the first class was that you had to be "lite" to do the aerobics. The slim, trim instructor told me (as she was giving me CPR) that I would do fine and to keep trying. She promised I would "get the hang of it." She convinced me to return the following week. I did, and I met with the same frustration and exhaustion. On week three, I quit.

Another exercise effort was an early morning walking group at a local mall. I joined with the hope of making new friends while exercising. I purchased suitable shoes, my first pair of walking shoes.

The next day I sleepily but enthusiastically arrived at the mall. The group members were already walking. I tried to join in, but I soon discovered I was definitely out of my league. These walkers really walked! They walked so fast I couldn't keep up with them. Over and over again, the walkers passed me by as they circled the interior of the mall. I slowed my already slow pace. If I couldn't keep up, I could at least do a little window shopping. I spent the remaining time looking at clothes I couldn't wear and things I couldn't afford to buy. What a depressing experience! At least, I rationalized, I wouldn't have to force myself out of bed in the wee hours of the morning, an unbearable effort for a non-morning person.

With this exercise failure came a treadmill. It was added to my unused exercise bike and an assortment of other "miracle" exercise equipment sold on late-night (my time of day) television for "just $19.95."

The treadmill would definitely be the answer to my lack of exercise. I placed it in the recreation room in front of the television. I could watch my favorite programs and exercise at the same time. I could walk, rain or shine, in the privacy of my home. This was the answer!

On day one I managed five minutes on the treadmill. The telephone rang and I just had to answer it (good excuse, huh!). I didn't return to the treadmill that day or in the days to come. I was just too busy.

Soon the treadmill became something to put things on, especially laundry baskets. I sometimes thought of it—how could I not? It was right there right in front of me—but I never got on it.

I'd find another way to exercise, but I never did . . . until I got the health club offer.

Now the health club was making me another offer I couldn't refuse. Having learned the benefits of exercise, I could share this knowledge with other overweight women.

I always thought I would have to lose weight first, get down to a more realistic size, before I could exercise. I know now that no matter what your size, no matter how overweight you are, you can and should exercise. With WOWS I can get this message out. I can make a difference, and I have. Over the past two years, almost one hundred women have joined the WOWS program. Many of these continue to work out on a regular basis. Like me, they have learned the importance of exercise in losing weight and getting fit. They have benefited from the support of a group, one that understands their specific problems. They have gone from woes to WOWS!

SUNDAY, SEPTEMBER 11, 1994

Today while I was watching a TV talk show I learned a few sayings that should help me with my program. One—"The mouth is the gateway to good health"—is really true. Now I put only good foods into my mouth (well, to be honest, every so often a forbidden cookie or a bite of cake or candy does get in), and this, combined with regular exercise, has resulted in better fitness. Another thing I learned was to say "Halt" and take a breather when I am hungry . . . angry . . . lonely . . . tired. It's at these times that I tend to get off the track and return to my old, unhealthy eating habits.

My 1,800-calorie food plan usually keeps me from feeling hungry. I try to calm down, breathe slowly, and say a few prayers to get rid of anger. If I get lonely—which luckily is hardly ever—I know some alone adults who would love a telephone call or visit. And I try to get the proper amount of sleep so I can avoid being tired.

Remembering and using the Halt principle can help us when we are tempted to overeat or when we crave unhealthy foods. But for many of us with weight problems, this simple technique is probably not enough.

I'm not a health expert and I don't know the complex reasons why some of us have weight problems while others do not. I do know that our weight problems are affected by such factors as biology (physical characteristics, genetics, family history), behavior (recurrent patterns and habits, responses to stimulation or environment), psychology (thoughts, attitude, mental state), and emotions (feelings). To lose weight you must learn how these factors impact you and how to change those you can.

You can't do much about genetics, but just because every female member of your family is overweight doesn't mean you have to be overweight. Eat less and exercise more to break this family trait. Be a trendsetter!

Changing your behavior can be one of the hardest things to do, but with effort and, more important, determination, it can be done. If you have a bowl of ice cream with topping every Saturday night for a treat, switch to fruit. If you wake up each day at 7 A.M., try waking up at 6:45 A.M. and spend fifteen minutes doing abdominal crunches or some other exercise. If you always stop at the doughnut shop on your way to work, take a different route so you won't be tempted. There are numerous ways to change our behavior that will help us stay on track, on our road to good health and fitness. With little modifications in our behavior will come success.

Behavior Modifications That Worked for Me

- *Make a food plan.* Plan what you are going to eat the next day, the next meal. A plan helped me stay in control.

- *Always sit down when you eat.* I discovered I did not pay attention to what I was eating when I stood or when I ate on the run. I also tended to eat more and to eat unhealthy foods. If you sit, you enjoy your food more.

- *Never eat while you are on the telephone.* Again, you are probably not paying attention to what or how much you're eating. I didn't when I was on the phone.

- *Don't eat while you're cooking, baking, or preparing a meal.* One little taste should do the trick if you need to test what you're preparing. You can take in a lot of calories by eating while you cook. If you are hungry, have a low-calorie, low-fat snack (lettuce salad, fruit) before you start cooking. Better yet, have a large glass of water.

- *Walk out of the kitchen if you're tempted by food.* Walk into another room and ask yourself if you really need to eat that food. Remind yourself that eating this food will not help you reach your goal.

- *Stay out of the kitchen whenever possible.* If you are away from food, you won't be tempted.

- *Don't eat anything out of a bag, box, or its original container.* Remove the correct portion, then put the package away. If you're like me, when you eat straight from the package, you probably don't stop until the supply runs out.

- *Always have good "filler foods" on hand for snacking.* Keep such foods as vegetable soup and salad fixings in the refrigerator. Reach for these when you need a snack.

- *Take a long, luxurious bath at night.* It can be your treat instead of snacking on food. Or find some other form of luxury.

- *Have an alternative plan for snacking.* If you have a food craving, you might go into your bedroom, get down on your knees, and ask God for help (this worked for me). Or, get down on the floor and do some crunches for your abs. (It's better to work on your tummy than to put extra food in it!)

We also need a positive mental attitude to go along with our behavior modifications. Without this positive mind-set, we will fail. Negative thoughts will cause roadblocks on our journey to good health and fitness. This is why we must always, every day and many times a day, tell ourselves we are worth good health. We are worthy of fitness. We deserve to be the best we can be. We must also tell ourselves that we can do it. We can achieve our goals, and we will!

Emotions play a pivotal role in causing our weight problems. Often, emotions prompt us to eat even when we are not hungry. We use our reactions to certain situations as excuses for overeating. We get a disturbing telephone call from our mother, our mother-in-law, a friend, the children's principal, a collection agency, and it sends us to the refrigerator and food to "make it better." We lose a job, our husband loses his job, we get a bill we didn't expect, our child brings home a failing report card. These alarming situations send us directly to our comfort foods—those foods that have in the past, and will now, make us feel better.

While I cannot guarantee that your journey, once you start,

will go smoothly—it hasn't for me—I have discovered that by managing my emotions, by turning to family and friends instead of food, I have been successful.

Anytime we use excuses, even though they are valid, we give ourselves permission to fail. Many unsuccessful dieters have used biological, behavioral, psychological, and emotional factors as their excuses. While we can't eliminate all of these factors, if we do a better job of controlling them, we can alleviate many of our eating problems. That's what I did!

FRIDAY, SEPTEMBER 16, 1994

My new lifestyle has resulted in another change. Because the foods I eat are so healthy and so low in fat, I can now sleep on only one pillow. For years I have been propped up on a minimum of two pillows, usually three. This is because almost nightly I had terrible heartburn. Sometimes I would have to get up in the middle of the night to vomit. Now I know it was my poor diet. I was eating too many fatty foods. Also, I ate too late at night. I used to live on antacid tablets. Now I get a peaceful night's sleep on one pillow.

SUNDAY, SEPTEMBER 18, 1994

I was looking at family pictures today, and I noticed there were very few with me in them. There's a reason for this. Fat people don't like to have their picture taken. They don't want a permanent, visible record of their weight problem.

I'll never forget my disappointment about eight years ago when we had a family portrait taken. I took great care to assure that we all looked nice for this family picture. The girls and I wore light blue tops; Andy and his dad wore navy blue vests over light blue shirts. We all looked wonderful. Everyone's hair was just perfect. It was going to be a great picture.

When the proofs arrived I couldn't have been more disappointed. The photographer had me seated on the left; my husband on the right. The children were basically scattered around my husband. The finished product found me taking up more than two thirds of the picture. The other four members of the family fit comfortably in the remaining one third. All the viewer could see was a "sea of blue," otherwise known as my chest. Even more disconcerting, the picture made me realize that I outweighed the rest of the family combined. If you added up my husband's weight and that of each of the children, I weighed more than the total.

THURSDAY, OCTOBER 6, 1994

This lifestyle change is hard. Some days I get so depressed because I have so far to go to get to my goal. Then I get mad at myself. I can't believe I let myself get to this enormous amount of weight. I am willing to stay on this Food Plan for Life (I have no choice), but I wish I could already be skinny. This slow but sure approach works, but I sure wish it wasn't going so slow! I wish I were rid of the excess weight now.

SUNDAY, OCTOBER 30, 1994

Hip! Hurray! I lost 7 pounds this month. This food plan and exercise are working!

THURSDAY, NOVEMBER 3, 1994—MY FIFTIETH BIRTHDAY

I have been depressed all week. I should be happy. I've lost 52 pounds for my fiftieth birthday. This is a great achievement, but I am still depressed. Even Family Circle's *pronouncement that I was "50 and Fabulous" didn't help.*

I have never had a problem with my age, but turning fifty has not been fun. I keep telling myself that I am healthier and more fit than

I have ever been, so much so that I have probably added years to my life. That in itself, I reckon, makes me younger than my fifty years. Logically, I can handle reaching this age, but emotionally, whew! I guess I never thought I'd be fifty years old.

The year has truly been one of major changes. Not only have I lost weight and learned the secret to lifelong health and fitness, but my baby Emily has moved out of elementary school into middle school (I've been in grade school for many years with three children) and Andy got his driving permit. We're all getting older and I'm taking the lead.

Turning fifty can be a crucial time in a person's life. It's an important mark on the lifeline. It represents an existence of half a century.

Some individuals, and you may be one of them, believe that when they reach the age of fifty, they should "settle" right where they are. They should accept themselves as they are, because they probably will never change. They believe, if they are overweight at fifty, and have been for years, that they will always be overweight. If they didn't lose weight in their twenties, thirties, or forties, what makes them think they will lose weight now? Why even try? What's the use?

But there is a good reason—lots of good reasons—to lose weight at any time, especially in the fifties. Losing weight will improve your quality of life now and in the years to come. It can decrease your chances of developing diseases such as diabetes, and it can lessen the likelihood of heart problems. It can help you avoid knee and hip replacement surgery. It can keep you out of a wheelchair, a nursing home, an early grave.

Getting fit is important at any age. Older individuals who become more active and eat healthy, including those with medical problems, may feel better and have more energy than ever before.

With all the benefits of exercise and maintaining a healthy weight, why would you want to "settle" and stay overweight? I wanted to be the best I could be. And it took being in my fifties to achieve this goal! No matter what your age, this, too, should be your goal!

SATURDAY, NOVEMBER 5, 1994

What a day! My husband surprised me with a birthday party—120 guests, a DJ, and a buffet dinner. He did great, and I was really surprised. When I walked into the party, the DJ played "Here She Comes, Miss America." When I was a child I always pretended that I was Miss America. I'd walk out between the sheets drying on the backyard clothesline and bow to my imaginary adoring audience. I'd sing in front of the sheets, then dance, then wave to the millions of Americans who were thrilled when the imaginary crown was placed on my head. Year after year after year I was Miss America. Although I was fat, I imagined that I was beautiful in the bathing suit and long gown (really my mother's old pink slip) contests. Tonight, when I walked into the party, I felt just as beautiful as the Miss America of my youth. The rest of the evening was wonderful as guests commented on my weight loss and told me how good I looked. I danced the night away with my Prince Charming, Tom. I guess fifty isn't so bad after all!

MONTH OF DECEMBER 1994

I blew it . . . royally! I had a terrible time keeping to my food plan all month. I used the holidays and the many (there were seventeen) parties as excuses for doing badly. I seemed to eat everything in sight.

I am really disappointed in myself. I thought I was in control. Al-though my food plan went out the window, I never wavered on exercise. No matter how busy I was, I managed to get in an hour of exercise most days. I praised myself for this success and vowed to work on the other leg—the food plan.

THURSDAY, JANUARY 5, 1995

Today's meeting with Dr. Wagner was very fruitful. I had many con-cerns and many questions. Why did I go overboard? Dr. Wagner said that years and years of bad eating habits (overeating and overin-dulging) can't be eliminated overnight, or even in a year. She re-minded me that although I did badly over the holidays, it was an improvement over previous holiday seasons. Also, I kept to my exer-cise program. I admitted that I gained weight (I said 2 pounds, but it was more like 10). She said it's not important what I ate during the holidays, but what I am going to do from now on.

Before I left our meeting I made a new resolve. I will succeed!

FRIDAY, JANUARY 20, 1995

Good week. I'm doing very well. Another WOWS session started. There are eight women in the class ranging in age from thirty-two to seventy-three years. These classes give me added enthusiasm for my personal project and for helping others. The women in my previous classes told me I not only inspired them, but I helped them get started on a good exercise and nutrition program. Because of me, they said, they will succeed.

TUESDAY, JANUARY 24, 1995

Tonight while I was in bed, I felt my thighs. They are still big, but they are now firmer. It felt good to touch them. I hardly ever looked at or touched my body before. Although I mentally felt like a woman, because of my great size, physically I never did. My body was just something to wash, cover, and get me around. Now I look at my body. My stomach is flat. My figure is becoming more defined. I'm beginning to like what I see! I am woman!

FRIDAY, JANUARY 27, 1995
Now I don't have to have the kids pick things up when I drop them. I can bend without much effort. It's little things like this that keep me motivated, that keep me going.

THURSDAY, FEBRUARY 2, 1995
I still dislike exercising, but I must admit I do love the way I feel. I now have a bounce to my step. I move fast when necessary and I can get up out of a low chair or couch easily. This is freedom. I wish other overweight people could feel the way I'm beginning to feel. I no longer feel as if I am handicapped.

One of the most distressing aspects of being obese is how excess weight can be a handicap to normal living. Being severely overweight prevented me from easily climbing steps to friends' front doors (someone always had to help me); from using regular stalls in public rest rooms (my girth fit only the handicap facilities); from getting down (I'd plop) and up (impossible without aid) from the ground.

A few years ago my husband surprised me with tickets to an outdoor symphony performance. We planned to take a picnic basket and a blanket and sit on a hill under the stars and listen to music. Tom was enthusiastic about our upcoming romantic evening. I was filled with dread.

The night arrived after an afternoon of trying on everything in my closet. I just didn't have "ground sitting" clothes. (You can't wear muumuu-type dresses when you're spread out on the ground.) I found some knit pants and a top that would have to do.

When we arrived at the concert we located a great spot on the hill, spread our blanket, and settled in (I ungracefully plopped down) for a night of music. Soon we were imprisoned by a mass of blankets filled with other picnickers and music lovers. Their closeness made me uncomfortable, as did the hard ground. I shifted. I wiggled. I turned one way, then the other. My great mass prevented me from achieving any comfort.

Halfway through the concert I realized I had to go to the bathroom. How could I get up and climb over our neighbors to make it to the rest room? I couldn't! I'd have to hold it. It was one of the most uncomfortable forty-five minutes of my life.

When the show was finally over, relief had to wait until everyone left. I didn't want anyone around to watch as Tom pulled me up from the ground. Finally the hill was clear. Tom, after much straining, pulled me to my feet. We rushed to the rest rooms. I didn't make it. I had waited too long. Our romantic evening was destroyed by my excess weight. I never felt so undignified, so despicable.

SATURDAY, FEBRUARY 11–SATURDAY, FEBRUARY 18, 1995
A week in San Diego for a family vacation. This would be a real test for me. I planned ahead of time that I would follow my food plan and I would exercise. And, although I had a few little failures, the week was marked mostly with success. I ate healthy most of the time and I exercised daily in the hotel's gym. Also, I walked for four hours through the San Diego Zoo with my family. I kept up with them and it wasn't a strain. I was beginning to feel I was part of life!

MONDAY, FEBRUARY 20, 1995

Got on the scale today to check vacation damage. There was none. I did not gain one pound on vacation. This is great success!

MONDAY, FEBRUARY 27, 1995

Two more women joined WOWS. One is extremely overweight. In addition, she recently lost her job and is afraid of looking for another because of her weight. She is giving herself six months to get into shape. I told her it's not good to put such limitations on herself. I believe you cannot set a time limit for weight loss. You have to adopt a slow but sure philosophy. If you set unrealistic deadlines, you will either resort to unhealthy dieting to meet the goal, or you will be severely disappointed if you don't lose the weight in the specified time. I am going to work with this woman to help her learn that consistent progress, not a deadline, is the best way to achieve success.

Chapter 8

Moving on Down!

Movement. That's what keeps me going.

Most of my adult life has been spent in pursuit of activities done from a sitting position—crafts, sewing, reading, writing, playing bridge. These were just a few of my favorite reposing endeavors. Even as a mother of small children, I was able to keep my buttocks comfortably at rest. A ranch-type (no steps) home and a fenced-in outdoor play area made for easy maintenance of active youngsters. Also, my husband, and sometimes friends, took care of the heavy-duty action.

One time when Andy, my son, was a toddler, he toddled out the front door and started running down the street. I tried to run after him, but he soon outdistanced me. A car was coming toward him. A neighbor—a slim, athletic woman—looked out her window and saw the tragedy about to take place in the street. She ran to Andy and scooped him up just seconds before the fast-moving car reached him. I, because of my weight, had been unable to catch up to my baby. My relief was mixed with the shame of knowing that I wasn't a fit mother. But did this move me to action? No! I hadn't yet reached that low place where enough was enough.

Movement didn't come until I started this program . . . and, boy, did it ever come into my life! Once I began to exercise, an amazing thing happened. I began to feel great! I began to know how a healthy body is supposed to feel.

Now that toddler I couldn't catch is a teenager and he has trouble keeping up with me. Recently I invited Andy to "power walk" at the high school track with me. This varsity athlete agreed and kept up with me for the first two miles. On mile three, he began to slow down. By mile four he was back in the car waiting for his mother to finish her rounds!

The legs aren't the only things moving these days. The marker on the scale has been steadily moving to the left. It's moved down to 250. That's a 60-pound weight loss, based on my *Family Circle* start. How triumphant!

During my journey I discovered that the word "triumph" is comprised of "tri" (try) and "umph" (oomph). I'm giving my all— my oomph—as I try to succeed. Because of this, I'm moving on down the road and down the scale!

FRIDAY, MARCH 3, 1995
Emily's (my baby) twelfth birthday. I had a small piece of cake and I didn't feel guilty. I've reconciled myself to the fact that I'll never be perfect, so an occasional lapse is okay as long as I plan for it, which I did. I cut down on breads (two) today to allow for this treat.

FRIDAY, MARCH 10, 1995
This week I noticed a few more reasons why weight loss (and being fit) is wonderful. I don't snore as much! This is because I have lost so much girth around my middle. Also, my migraines have been greatly

reduced in number. Healthy food and exercise, which help reduce stress, are, I am sure, responsible for this.

MONDAY, MARCH 13, 1995

I exercise six days a week without fail. I can't believe I am so consistent. Consistent. *Now there's a word that marks all success. If you consistently eat a low-fat, low-calorie diet, you will lose weight. If you consistently exercise, you get fit. I am consistent with exercise. I will try to be more consistent with my food plan.*

THURSDAY, MARCH 30, 1995

I was looking in the mirror today at my double chin. (It was a triple!) I can't believe that I ever had "chin bulk" because this is one area of my body that I always exercised—eating and talking. Maybe my double chin is really a muscle!

SATURDAY, APRIL 1, 1995

April Fool's Day! I would be a real fool to blow it now that I have come so far. Unfortunately, some days I say "the hell with it" and eat everything in sight. Then, of course, I feel guilty.

I had always been a closet eater. I hid my eating problems because, heaven forbid, I didn't want anyone to think I was responsible for my fat. I liked to believe, and have everyone else believe, that my fat came on by magic, with no help from me. It couldn't be what I ate! I ate only small portions of the right foods! Right?

So I ate secretly, when and where no one was around. There is one thing that nobody, ever, has seen me do. I have never eaten an ice cream cone walking down the street. I never wanted passersby to think "What is that fat girl/woman doing eating an ice cream cone?" Instead, I bought a half gallon of ice cream and ate the whole thing when I was home alone. I then hid the evidence, the empty carton, in the bottom of the garbage. I did this with other foods, too. Bags of chips, bags of cookies, whole cakes, a dozen doughnuts. But I did this only in secret—in the closet.

Now I am out of the closet, at least most of the time!

FRIDAY, APRIL 14, 1995
Many individuals have no idea what it is like to be fat, really fat. They have never been faced with the embarrassment of not being able to fit into a chair, an airline seat, a theater seat.

During my fat life I have broken two toilet seats (one at my house; one at a friend's) and numerous chairs. Luckily, most of these chairs were ours. However, one, a flimsy director-style chair, resulted in the loss of a freelance writing job.

I was in the middle of an interview with the head of an advertising agency. The interview was going well. The president seemed impressed with my credentials. Then it happened. First there was a terrible cracking sound. Then I was on the floor. After checking to see if I was hurt, the interviewer kindly assured me not to worry. "These chairs aren't very sturdy," he said. However, I didn't "fall" into this job. I never heard from the agency again.

My excess weight was also responsible for couch damage (the springs) and, sadly, for the destruction of our four-poster bed, a wedding present we gave each other.

Over the years I noticed that my side of our queen-size bed was slanting toward the floor. It got so bad that one night I felt I was going to roll off the bed. Tom and I got up to check what was causing the problem. It was the metal frame. My excess weight had, with time, severely bent the frame. I was so embarrassed. My wonderful husband said it probably wasn't my fault. He said the frame wasn't very strong so it could have happened to anyone. Then why wasn't his side of the bed bent?

TUESDAY, APRIL 25, 1995

I have really progressed in my fitness quest. In my former life, if I strayed from my diet I would just keep straying. After all, I reasoned, I must be a terrible, awful person if I couldn't stick to the diet. Besides, since I goofed, I would tell myself, there is nothing I can do about it now. I've wrecked the whole day, so I might as well eat whatever I want. Now if I stray, I feel bad for a few minutes, then I get right back on my food plan. I don't wait until the next meal, the next day, the next week. I get back on track immediately.

WEDNESDAY, MAY 10, 1995

I am faster than an automatic sliding door! For years I have gone to my doctor's office and walked in from the outside through the sliding door. It always opened just as I reached it. Today I walked right into the door. I was walking so fast, the door didn't have time to open. I was really startled, but as I rubbed my bumped head I started laughing. I now walk so fast that some things can't keep up with me.

I also have a zip to my step. For years I waddled very slowly to my destinations. It was as if I had the weight of the world on my shoulders. That's one-third right! I did have the weight, but it wasn't the world's and it wasn't only on my shoulders. It was mine and it was also on my hips, chin, legs, arms, stomach, just about everyplace! And while some is still there, some has vanished. My load is getting lighter and so is my step!

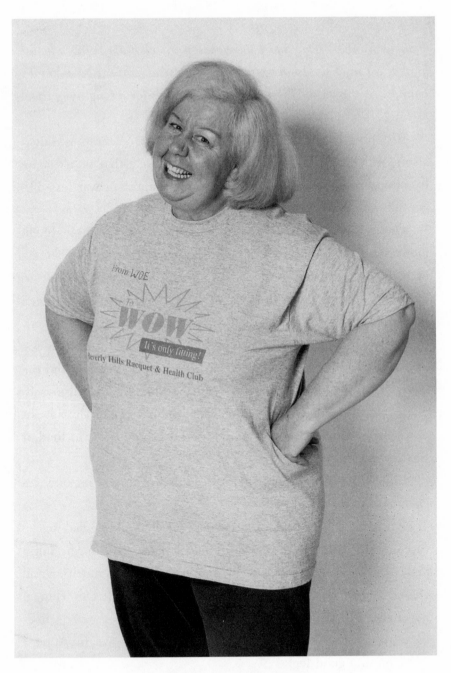

Dressed to lead my WOWS class.

MAUREEN ELECTA MONTE

SUNDAY, MAY 14, 1995

Today is Mother's Day and I have reason to celebrate being a better mother for my kids. I have reached the halfway point. I have lost 75 pounds. At this rate, I'll be around for my kids for a long, long time!

Reaching the halfway point was cause for celebration, but it also marked the beginning of a downward cycle that didn't abate for almost a month. I began to rest on my laurels. I was less diligent about following my food plan.

One reason for this was that I had worked so hard for eighteen months and had *only* achieved a 75-pound weight loss. I, like everybody else, know individuals who go on diets and are able to drop 100 pounds in less than a year. My 75 pounds in eighteen months was, to me, no big deal. I looked in the mirror and saw only a heavy woman who needed to lose weight. I couldn't see anything else. I felt I had failed the *Family Circle* readers and the many others who were counting on me. I felt I had failed myself.

I started eating everything in sight. I didn't care if it was high- or low-fat. I didn't care how many calories it had. If it was food, it was for me!

Also, I began smoking cigarettes here and there, but only socially and only with friends.

Eating and smoking. My former bad habits seemed to be catching up with me. I was eating like a pig. (Well, maybe not a pig, but at least a piglet! My eighteen months of good nutrition and changed lifestyle didn't allow me to go whole hog!) One thing I never gave up was exercise. I continued my six-days-a-week schedule at top intensity. And this helped me to not gain weight. At least I was on one good leg!

Friday, June 23, 1995

How do you stay motivated? How do you stay on track? According to Dr. Wagner, the best motivation is to look at what I've accomplished. So now I have what I call assess my success times throughout the week. If I feel weak and tempted, I go over in my mind all those small things I can now do, such as walking up stairs, climbing the stepladder, that I couldn't do when I weighed more than 300 pounds.

Ways to Finish Your Journey

- *Be patient.* Don't expect overnight miracles. It took time, maybe even years, for you to get physically unfit. It will take time and effort for you to get fit.
- *Think one meal at a time—one day at a time—one pound at a time. Go slow but sure.*
- *Relapses are part of life.* Most attempts at change don't work on the first try. If you have a relapse, don't berate yourself. Try to learn from your mistakes and then get right back on your food plan and exercise program.
- *Give yourself permission to occasionally eat and enjoy appropriate amounts of your favorite foods.* Total deprivation can lead to bingeing on bad foods.
- *Don't skip meals.* If you do, you'll be more tempted to overeat at a later time.
- *Think positive.* You can choose the attitude you want to embrace. If you believe you can succeed, you will.
- *Don't use past or present circumstances as an excuse to eat inappropriately.*
- *Avoid self-pity.* It destroys character, weakens your re-

solve, and it definitely doesn't endear you to those around you.

- *Trust yourself.* Self-trust is the secret to success.
- *Reward yourself when you reach "mini goals"—5, 10, 25 pounds.* Having a manicure is a nice treat to celebrate a 10-pound weight loss; a massage, facial, or other beauty treatment can mark 25 pounds. (When I lost 50 pounds, I treated myself to two down-filled feather pillows. Each night, as my head slowly sinks into these luxurious acquisitions, I'm reminded of my weight-loss success.)
- *If you are having a difficult time, recite the Serenity Prayer.*

    God, grant me the serenity

    To accept the things I cannot change,

    The courage to change the things I can,

    And the wisdom to know the difference.

SUNDAY, JUNE 25, 1995

I have become agile and flexible because of exercise. My body has become more than just a carrier. It's becoming a prized possession.

I will continue to do the exercise that can help guarantee fitness. I know that what I do now can help determine what I will be like during my senior years.

FRIDAY, JUNE 30, 1995

I had to purchase brownies for the girls in Emily's baton competition. I went to the Sara Lee Outlet for these and a number of other items, primarily bagels. I didn't notice that the store had a "special," a free cheesecake with the purchase of a certain number of items. As I was putting my purchases away this evening, the cheesecake—my greatest food obsession—fell out of the bag. Temptation set in. One small piece wouldn't hurt. So I had one, then two, then the entire cake! (I couldn't leave any evidence of my failure for the family to discover. And I couldn't throw this precious booty in the garbage. So I was forced to eat the whole thing!) Besides, I didn't ask for this cheesecake! I didn't buy it! It must have been manna from heaven!

After stuffing the cake into my mouth, I felt awful. I was disappointed with myself, plus my stomach ached. I felt I was going to throw up. Unfortunately, I didn't. Instead I was awake most of the night taking antacid tablets. It was then that I realized the cheesecake wasn't a gift from God, but a present from Sara Lee. And she certainly was a "friend" I needed to avoid!

Sunday, July 2, 1995

Friends had our family over for dinner to celebrate the holiday weekend. What was to be a pleasant time didn't turn out that way. The wife, a good friend of mine, is constantly complaining that she and her husband need to lose weight. (And they do!) However, although she knows how hard I am trying to achieve my goal, she chose to serve pizza (double cheese, thank you), spareribs, numerous fat-filled accompaniments, and for dessert, strawberry shortcake. She served not one thing that would be considered low-fat and/or healthy. By her words and actions, I had the feeling she was trying to see if I really could be good. Also, I believe that she, like a number of others, wants me to stay fat. After all, I was always bigger than most and heaven forbid, I better not get smaller than them!

This dinner was definitely a sabotage maneuver. However, it didn't work. I was very good. I ate one small—the smallest—piece of pizza; passed on all the other fat-filled items; chose only strawberries for dessert, no cake, no whipped topping.

My friend marveled at my self-control. "You're soooo good," she enthused. However, I think she was disappointed because I didn't "break" once during the hundreds of times that evening when she tried to get me to eat more.

Sabotage! This is one of the biggest problems dieters face when undertaking a program like mine. And it comes from a multitude of sources. In my case, the sabotage has come from friends who don't want me to succeed: the overweight ones who don't want me to leave them, the slim ones who don't want me to join them!

Sometimes, the sabotage has come from my husband, who, I believe, on some level doesn't want things to change. And he does have some reason to feel this way. During our marriage, in the midst of fights, I have threatened to leave him "when I lose the weight." In my mind, this was a frivolous threat voiced in the heat of the argument. However, with Tom, these words stuck.

One time, early in my marriage, my mother said, "Sandra, if you don't lose weight, you're going to lose Tom!" She said this in front of my husband, who was tired of my mother's picking on my weight. "Mom," he said, "I don't want Sandra to lose weight!" My mother looked at Tom as if he were nuts. He continued, "You know, Mom, I'm afraid Sandra would leave me if she lost weight!"

On the ride home, I asked Tom if he really thought I would leave him if I were slim. He said he did. I reassured him a number of times that I would never, ever leave him. "You will never leave me?" he asked. *"Never!"* I said. He then got a twinkle in his eye. "Then, if you will never leave me, lose weight," he said. We both laughed. However, Tom's insecurity continues, although on a smaller scale, even today.

Subversion also came from me. Although I have always wanted to shed the excess weight, or thought I did, I believe that, on a subconscious level, I really was afraid of being slim. After all, I have been able to hide for all these years in a very thick shell.

I was comfortable with my large body. The relationships I have were formed while I was in this cocoon of fat. I like who I am now. What if the new package alters my personality? What if I change and become a person I don't like, one who isn't likable?

It's been said that heavy people "try harder" and "are funnier" because of their weight. They have to make up for being "outside the norm." Maybe I became so friendly as a child because I was fat, or maybe I was this way because it was really me. I don't know the answer to this, and, at times, I am afraid. When I'm slender will I continue to reach out to all kinds of people? Will I have empathy for heavy individuals? Or will I feel that I'm better than others?

I hope only the body changes, and not the person I am.

Another major source of sabotage came from my mother and sisters. Although I come from a loving family (I have three sisters), we are not immune to the normal rivalry and jealousy found in most close units.

Two of my sisters also have a weight problem, although never to the extent of mine. When I started my program they were very excited for me and hopeful for my success. They wanted me to help them in their weight-loss struggles by sharing the nutritional information I received and learned. I did, but they weren't ready to use it. They hadn't reached the point where enough is enough.

When I began losing weight, my sisters said very little about what I was doing and rarely asked how it was going. When they saw me at family functions, they rarely told me how good I looked. It was as if my weight-loss/fitness program didn't exist.

As I began to achieve even more success, they also changed

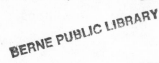

their cooking habits. When they had me over for dinner after I first started the food plan, they were careful to serve foods that were healthy, low-fat, and low in calories. But as the pounds began to come off, their meals changed to the wrong foods, such as chicken in sauces, potato salad, and, of course, my real tempter—cheese-cake. They no longer encouraged my success.

My mother often sided with my sisters. For years she had told me she was worried about my health. She even cried at times when she told me she feared I would die because I was so heavy and unhealthy. Now that I was successful, she hardly took notice, especially in the presence of my sisters.

My size 10 sister, the only one of the four of us who has always maintained a healthy weight, said Mom didn't say anything about how well I was doing because she didn't want my two overweight sisters to feel bad. Also, according to my trim sister, my success only made my other sisters feel even worse about their weight. I understood how they felt . . . I'd been there, for so many years I was there!

So how do I deal with sabotage?

When I go to gatherings with family and friends, I always bring foods that are part of my plan for me to eat and to share with others. At one family function, I was asked to bring a cheesecake. I did, but I also brought a fresh fruit salad for those, like me, who needed a healthy alternative.

I no longer ask for compliments on my slimmer looks. I keep my mouth shut and if they come, I say "thank you." If they are not offered, I go to the nearest mirror, look at myself, and mentally praise my success.

Also, I have had long talks with my husband and children to assure them that, although my body is changing, my feelings for them are just as strong, if not stronger, than before. I continue to ask for their support. I remind them that certain foods tempt me and ask them, if possible, to keep those foods out of the house. They try to eat "the junk" away from home and stick to healthy choices in my presence.

My own sabotage has been a little more difficult to deal with. Ever since I was a child, I saw myself as a beautiful princess, or movie star . . . anyway, I saw myself as famous and beautiful and, more important, *slender.* With the weight loss, I was getting closer to my long-held dreams of being, if not beautiful, then at least slender. As I got closer to my dreams, I seemed to up the sabotage. But with resolve and some good talks with myself, I have been able to limit this self-destructive behavior. I have decided it's time I played a starring role, instead of being lost in the chorus. I work every day to achieve reality and not just be the princess of my dreams. And that's what it takes. *Work!*

Chapter 9

Help!

You can get real comfortable resting on your laurels. At least, I did! Even though I wished it were more, achieving a 75-pound weight loss was a remarkable feat for me. Once before I had reached the midpoint in a diet program. However, then I gave up and gained all the weight back and then some.

Now I had a real task before me. I had to go beyond the half-way point and reach the finish line. I had to stay focused. However, I was having a tough time.

FRIDAY, AUGUST 11, 1995

Tonight I went to dinner with my sisters and mom. We were scheduled to go to one restaurant that offered lots of good food selections. Instead, because one of my sisters was so insistent, we ended up at a Chinese place. The group then wanted to order the meal for five. Although unhappy with this selection, I agreed. I should have been stronger and insisted that I couldn't eat Chinese (too fatty, and MSG is bad for my migraines), but I went along with the group. I like to please people too much, and, because of this, I ended up paying with my head and stomach!

Pleasing people! That seems to be our duty as women. Sometimes, in the process of fulfilling this role, we limit ourselves . . . we sabotage our own best interests.

The only way I have been able to achieve success is by being selfish. At times, I have to say "no" to friends. And—this is a hard one—I must say "no" to my husband and children when my needs are not in sync with theirs.

In my pre-program life, I was a willing volunteer in our community. Everyone at the kids' schools, at church, at the village offices, at the swim club knew they could call Mrs. Prysby if help was needed. I offered my time; I gave my efforts to all sorts of causes.

However, I learned almost from the beginning of my project that I just didn't have the time; I just couldn't give the effort. I learned, and this was very difficult for a "pleasing person," to discard those activities that didn't bring rewards. While I try never to cheat my family, I'm not so diligent in other areas. I need at least two hours a day for exercise. I need time to shop and to prepare healthy foods.

To make this time I have eliminated lots of "just chitchat" telephone calls. I have lowered my already low cleaning standards. I have put aside numerous unimportant tasks that formerly cluttered my life.

In order to streamline my body, I have organized my life. This decision has caused some family members (not Tom and the kids, they've been true supporters!) and friends to say I've "changed."

I've heard that some believe I'm not as "nice" as I used to be. What they are really saying is that I am not as available to do the things *they want*.

I *have* changed, not only in body, but in mind. I'm more mindful of my needs. I've learned to please myself!

THURSDAY, AUGUST 24, 1995
I have been busy most of the month working on my high school class reunion. Planning to attend a class reunion can really be a stressful time. I worried about my looks; I worried if people would be shocked at my weight; I worried if the cute, popular ones would still be cute and "stuck up." I worried that I would have a miserable time. And as I worried, I ate.

Why do we spend so much of our lives worrying about such superficial things? Why does how we look have such an impact on whether or not we have a good time?

Being involved in the reunion renewed memories of my school years. One in particular came to mind.

When I was in the second grade I had a friend named Diane. She was small and petite with blond hair and blue eyes. As cute as she was, her best feature, which I appreciated even as a seven-year-old, was her personality. She knew how to have fun, and I really liked being with Diane.

At this time, as at most times in my life, I was big. I was tall in size and wide in width. My mother said Diane and I looked "funny" together. We "looked strange together," she said, because we were "so disproportionate." She harped on this so much that I gave up my friendship with Diane. Even as a little child, I worried about what people would think. I let appearance win.

Appearance also won during other stages of my life. I chose

slim, trim friends over those with weight problems. I didn't want any observer to see me with another fat person and think, "Birds of a feather flock together." I thought if I was hidden in a sea of skinnies, nobody would realize I was fat.

How awful of me! I chose people because of their physical size, not their real substance. Luckily, as I matured—something I am still doing—I have learned to move beyond face (body) value. I have stopped worrying about what people think, which I did so often in my earlier years.

SUNDAY, AUGUST 27, 1995

My reunion weekend was filled with food, food, and more food. What a great time I had (and not because of the food). It was wonderful renewing old friendships and sharing stories of the past. It was also nice getting rave reviews from my former classmates. (Many were aware of my progress from reading Family Circle.)

I'd like to say I was perfect on my food plan, but I can't. Enough said?

SUNDAY, SEPTEMBER 10, 1995

Boy, have I been gliding. After I reached my 75-pound weight loss this summer, I went into neutral. I still exercise almost every day, but most times I don't think about what I am putting into my mouth. I've talked with Dr. Wagner and others and they say this is normal. But I don't want to hear it. I don't want permission to glide, and then slide. I want to lose the rest of this weight, so I want everyone to tell me what a "bad girl" I am. I have to turn this thing around. I have to get back on the road. I may even have gained weight, but I'm not getting on the scale to check. That could really depress me. I need to get more resolve and, more important, I need some higher help. I need God's help. Sometimes this project seems so monumen-

tal. I feel that I can't do it alone. I know I have lots of human help, but I also need spiritual intervention. With God's help, I'll do it!

Eureka! School is back in session and our family is back on schedule. Set schedules make it easier to stay on track. Vacations and other interruptions are real killers when it comes to this self-improvement program. These disruptions are something I have yet to conquer, but, with the grace of God, I will!

FRIDAY, SEPTEMBER 15, 1995

Met with Dr. Wagner today and she, as always, was a great help. I told her how very hard it is for me to get rid of foods that are not on my plan. For instance, a friend brought over a chocolate cake for the kids earlier this week. (I think she feels I'm depriving them!) They each took a piece, and although they liked it, the rest remained in the refrigerator for two days without any takers. For two whole days, each time I opened the refrigerator it called out to me. Although I usually don't eat chocolate (I get migraines), this chocolate cake kept beckoning me, hour after hour after hour. Finally, it was too much. I dug into it, really dug in. I ate most of the frosting and half the cake in less than fifteen minutes. Then I felt miserable. I felt like a pig and I worried that I would be struck by a world-class migraine. (Luckily, I wasn't!) I certainly took a giant step backward.

Dr. Wagner told me the garbage disposal is my friend. (She said the garbage can can be an enemy. It's too easy to retrieve forbidden food from the garbage can.) I told her I should have put the cake in the freezer. "No," she said. If the kids didn't eat this food right away, they weren't going to eat it later. I would be the one eating it later. "Put it down the garbage disposal" was her decree.

I told her I just couldn't throw away good food, especially with all the starving people in the world. (I sure did take my mom's words to heart when she tried to get me to clean my plate as a child.)

"Forget the starving people," said Dr. Wagner. "You couldn't take the cake to them anyway!" Then she offered another solution. Take the leftover cake to a nearby family with children. A family who would appreciate it. If I didn't know such a family, then I must learn to use the garbage disposal.

SATURDAY, SEPTEMBER 23, 1995

This program has taught me that I can no longer eat the foods I enjoyed in my pre-healthy days. I now make low-fat foods, but I don't try to duplicate what I ate before. I create new recipes with new tastes. For instance, I used to make tuna and potato salad with lots and lots of mayonnaise. When I tried tuna with the low-fat and no-fat salad dressing, it tasted awful. I couldn't eat it.

Now I have a new tuna salad. I use such ingredients as onion powder, no-fat sour cream and no-fat salad dressing (half and half), lots of celery (like before), but I also add green and/or red peppers (unlike before). It really tastes good and I have reduced the fat content.

For potato salad, I use only the white part of the hard-boiled egg and I make a dressing of half no-fat sour cream, half no-fat salad dressing. I add all the other ingredients—potatoes, celery, green pepper, onion. My former potato salad is transformed into a healthy dish.

So the secret, at least for me, to healthy cooking is create, don't try to duplicate! It works, my taste buds are getting new treats, and I'm adding healthy foods to my recipe files. It's fun creating new dishes, and it doesn't take a lot of time. It just requires a little experimenting.

MONDAY, OCTOBER 30, 1995

I am not being perfect on my program. I have found a number of excuses—fights with my husband, difficult teens, not enough sleep—for overeating and making poor food choices. I really haven't totally lost my focus. It's just that there are times when the focus is a bit fuzzy!

FRIDAY, NOVEMBER 3, 1995

Happy fifty-first birthday. My children surprised me with a very large, fattening dessert while at a restaurant to celebrate this special day. I should have passed on this dessert, but I didn't want to disappoint the givers. So I ate the whole thing, every one of those 2,000 calories. Would I have hurt their feelings if I didn't eat this dessert? Why didn't I offer to share it with them? Why do I still use special occasions as excuses for going off my food plan? I really have some work ahead of me if I am going to complete this journey. I must get stronger and I must learn to say "no."

SATURDAY, NOVEMBER 11, 1995

When I get depressed, which, fortunately, isn't too often, I still turn to food, the wrong kind of food. An apple just doesn't do it! My comfort foods are ice cream with butterscotch sauce, potato chips and dip, any kind of beef or pork with fat on it, and, my most beloved, cheesecake. I feel I deserve such treats. I know all about the psychological aspects of food. I know that certain foods represent happy times, security, even love. I know this and I shouldn't fall into the trap. But I do! I must look at what is causing the problem(s) and learn to solve it (them) with something other than food, such as talking to friends, exercise. Find a likable substitute. That's the solution.

MONDAY, NOVEMBER 20, 1995

Tom lost his job today. This is the third job this year. He needs help. I want him to get tested for Attention Deficit Disorder (ADD). He has all the classic symptoms. He doesn't stay focused; he doesn't finish anything. He says he is afraid of getting tested. "What if there isn't anything wrong with me? What if I'm just stupid?" said my electrical engineer husband. He isn't stupid. He's one of the brightest individuals I know . . . but he has to know this! He agreed to think about testing.

I thought I was over my depression, but this job loss has really set me back. No job just before the holidays! I can't believe it. This also means we lose our health insurance again for a while. With three kids this is devastating.

WEDNESDAY, NOVEMBER 22, 1995

Tom's job loss has really affected my program. I just don't care. I am so angry at him and I feel so sorry for myself. I bought a pack of cigarettes. I thought maybe smoking would help. It didn't. I feel awful physically and mentally. I went out and picked up a cheese-cake—my old standby. That didn't work either. I am so disgusted with myself for my transgressions. But right now I really don't care about anything.

THURSDAY, NOVEMBER 23, 1995

Thanksgiving Day. It will be okay . . . it will be okay . . . it will be okay. I keep saying this over and over again. If I say it enough maybe I'll believe it. Tom will get a new job. I'll be successful on my program. Tom will get tested for ADD and be put on medication. I won't sneak either of the Big Cs (cheesecake and cigarettes) any-more. Everything will be okay.

We went to one of my sisters—the supportive one—for dinner.

She usually serves foods that are on my food plan, but not today! Her dishes were, for the most part, extremely fattening. I really don't know why she did this. I guess everyone, including me, can get off to a good start but lose interest along the way. She used to be aware of my health needs, especially since her husband also needs to lose weight. Oh well. My program is not her problem. It's mine. I have to accept responsibility for it, and I have to make food choices and make sure there are foods I can eat.

I did do something really positive, something I have never done on Thanksgiving before. After dinner, at which I ate small servings, my sister and I went for a three-mile walk in the cold and in my uncomfortable dress shoes. The walk did me good and I was really proud of myself.

Walking has become my great stabilizer. It helps to keep me on my road, even when I'm not totally honest with my food choices.

You, too, need to discover how a regular walking program brings rewards with every step.

Consider this: Half an hour at five miles per hour—that's twelve minutes per mile—burns 265 calories. For me, the brisk walk on Thanksgiving Day took care of the piece of pumpkin pie with whipped topping that I just couldn't resist.

Walking is one of the best, and easiest, ways to fitness. And there's nothing to learn. We all know how to walk!

Walking is also easier on our joints than running or jogging. It doesn't put as much stress on our feet. (Besides, a brisk walk can burn more calories than jogging because, when we walk, we take more steps and use our arms more.)

There are other benefits from walking. One of the best is that this exercise can help us lose weight. Studies have shown that individuals who begin walking on a regular basis (four or more

days a week; half an hour at a time) can lose weight without alter-
ing their diet. If they combine this with a healthy eating plan, they
do even better.

In addition, according to research, walking can improve our
HDL or "good" cholesterol, and lower blood pressure. This means
walking just might help us live longer.

However, and this is important, you must be consistent. One
day here and one day there just won't do it. You must walk at least
two miles (four days is good; six is better) at a fairly fast pace (a
fifteen-minute mile) to achieve the maximum benefit.

THE MONTH OF DECEMBER 1995

*I am covering the whole month in this journal entry because, for the
most part, the whole month was a wash. I did terrible on my food
plan.*

*The loss of Tom's job, little money for holiday gifts and Libby's
birthday on the fifteenth, and the normal stress that comes with this
time of year made for one of the worst periods of time since I began
the program. I didn't worry about what I ate. (One reason is that I
had to buy cheap foods, which are not necessarily good foods.) About
the only things I did do right were continuing to exercise at least six
days a week and meeting with Dr. Wagner so I wouldn't go too far off
my road.*

*However, my program seemed to be the least of my concerns this
month. Am I using the current situation as an excuse? I don't know
the answer to that. I just know that, right now, my goal seems unattainable and, more stressing, unimportant.*

*But things didn't turn out as badly as I anticipated at the begin-
ning of the month. Libby did have a birthday party. I had a 50
percent off coupon at the Sara Lee (there's my friend again) Outlet,
so I purchased eight different cakes at a very reasonable price. I*

invited twenty of her friends for dessert, got out the crystal and china, lit lots of candles, and a great time was had by all. Of course, I had a piece, some big and some small, of most of the cakes. Now how is that for willpower!

Christmas also proved successful, even though there weren't many presents. I cried a few nights because of the meager Christmas, but the kids were thrilled with everything they got. They're a real blessing.

My optimism was beginning to return toward month's end and with it my desire to succeed. I just knew everything would be fine. I was ready to go forward.

Stress, if we let it get the best of us, can do terrible things to us. It can, as it did during this period of my program, eliminate motivation and impede progress.

Coping with stress is one of the most important factors in achieving weight loss. Exercise helps, but it can't overcome all the stress. If I was going to complete this project, I had to learn to cope with stress. If you, like me, can acquire coping skills, you can, like me, complete your journey.

Ways to Cope with Stress

- **Pray to God.**
- **Anticipate needs and plan ahead.**
- **Believe in yourself.**
- **Visualize winning.**
- **Review goals and/or make new ones.**
- **Know and meet your needs.**
- **Get in touch with your feelings.**
- **Set priorities.**

- Unclutter your life.
- Say "no" more often.
- Break down large tasks.
- Delegate tasks to others.
- Ask for help.
- Do things in moderation.
- Consider problems as challenges.
- Look at challenges as opportunities for success.
- Avoid negative people.
- Avoid negative thoughts.
- Stop talking negatively.
- Schedule quiet time for contemplation.
- Meditate.
- Think today—not tomorrow—is better!
- Smile.
- Work on your sense of humor, or develop one.
- Talk less and listen more.
- Breathe slowly.
- Stretch your limits, or just stretch.
- Cut down or eliminate caffeine beverages.
- Get enough sleep.
- Add a new exercise to your program.
- Complete a needed task.
- Break a bad habit.
- Do something new.
- Schedule playtime.
- Do something special with your child, husband, friend, family member.
- Ask for a hug.
- Call or visit a lonely person.
- Tell your friends how important they are to you.

- Say something nice to someone each and every day.
- Praise others.
- Praise yourself.
- Turn on music and sing or dance, or just listen and enjoy.
- Say "hello" to a stranger.
- Enjoy something beautiful in nature.
- Buy yourself a flower or a whole bunch.
- Look at and smell a flower.
- Read a book, a poem, or reread a favorite letter.
- Try a crossword puzzle, draw a picture, write a story, start a new craft or hobby.
- Light a candle.
- Take a bubble bath.
- Remember, only go one day at a time.
- RELAX!

These fifty-two coping suggestions can be used during difficult situations. Also, to achieve more peace in your life, pick out and practice one or a combination each week for a year. The more you use them, the more they will become part of your everyday life. They become your passport to success.

Chapter 10

Richard,
the Rescuer!

E nter 1996. I wasn't doing well on my program as the new year hit. My motivation and resolve were faltering. Over the past months I had been less diligent. I couldn't seem to get beyond the midpoint (75 pounds) of my 150-pound weight-loss goal. I needed help.

MONDAY, JANUARY 15, 1996

I know I must plan what I am going to eat the next day and I must write down what I do eat. This food diary will lead to success. However, I just don't do it. I just don't keep an accurate account of my food consumption. A member of my WOWS class offered a solution. She, too, had trouble planning and writing down her foods. Now she uses Richard Simmons' Deal-A-Meal program. It's designed with cards listing foods by groups (bread, protein, vegetables, etc.). You set up the cards based on your food plan on one side of a folder. When you eat a certain food, you move the card to the other side. This

WOWS member said the program is really helping her keep track of her food intake. She got one for me as a gift. I'll use it.

Using the Deal-A-Meal plan made me think of its creator, Richard Simmons. Now there was a person who knew all about motivation and keeping individuals on track. And, as everyone knew, he did his thing in a delightful, fun way. Maybe he could help me. It was time for another letter.

> *January 17, 1996*
> *Dear Richard:*
>
> *I know that everyone who writes you starts off: "I need your help!" I hate to start this letter the same way, but I do need your input.*
>
> *Now . . . what's my problem! Richard, I'm fizzling out! I'm losing my motivation. I'm resting on my laurels. And, since I have 75 pounds yet to lose and I have a lifetime ahead of me of healthy eating and exercise,* Help!
>
> *Please share with me some secrets for success. Also, please give me some motivational tips . . . I need inspiration.*
>
> *I hate imposing on you, especially when I have been given so much, but I need some of your sunshine.*
>
> > *Thank you.*
> > *Most sincerely,*

The minute I put the letter in the mail, I made an important decision. I wouldn't wait to hear from Richard to do something. (Besides, maybe I wouldn't hear from him. Little did I know that *Family Circle* was going to call and ask him to help me.) I would continue on my journey *now*. And I would progress well. After all, I knew what it took, and *I would do it!*

Long ago I had realized that if I wanted something accomplished, I'd have to do it myself. I couldn't depend on others to do the things I wanted done.

If you think about it, you, too, have learned this lesson. How many times have you asked the kids to clean their rooms, and how many times have you ended up doing it yourself? Then there are those tasks we ask our husbands to complete. How many of these do we take care of ourselves?

It's not just our families who fail to come through with help. In all areas of our lives we find that we can't always depend on others. We learn we often have to do things ourselves. This is also true when it comes to our personal weight-loss program.

Why would losing weight be any different? Sure, experts can offer assistance, but if we want to complete *our* goals, we have to take responsibility and *do the work!* I was willing to continue the work, with or without Richard Simmons!

FEBRUARY 1, 1996
To test the strength of my resolve, I will stay away from sweets for this whole month. All sweets!

FEBRUARY 18, 1996
Even though there are ice cream, cookies, and other goodies in the house, so far I haven't had one sweet. I am so proud of myself, and, more important, I know my goal is within reach.

I continue to use visualization and see myself in my soon-to-be body with a big smile on my face. I also dream about the future me. I have this dream that will someday come true.

MY DREAM

I walk into a large ballroom on the arm of my husband. There are steps down to the dance floor where hundreds (make that thousands) of people are congregated. I am wearing a black slinky floor-length dress with sheer netting on the long tight sleeves and at the neckline. It's simple but elegant. My white hair is perfectly coiffed and I have simple pearl earrings on and a single strand of pearls around my neck. My husband is handsome in his tuxedo.

The minute we walk into the room, each and every person on the ballroom floor looks up in our direction. All talking stops. There is not a sound in the room, just appreciative eyes coming my way from all the men. Then there is a collective "Ahhhhhhhhhh." Each and every woman in the room is jealous of how wonderful I look; each and every man is jealous of my husband, the man on my arm! My husband is so proud of my success; I'm so proud of my accomplishment. Tom and I spend the rest of the evening dancing the night away . . . with eyes only for each other!

SUNDAY, FEBRUARY 18–SATURDAY, FEBRUARY 24, 1996
This week I started something that really shouldn't be part of a good food plan. I decided to do the Cabbage Soup Diet, the one that is sweeping the nation. (Doesn't this sound like days of old when I tried just about everything to lose weight?) However, I'm not doing this strenuous diet to lose weight. It's a head thing! I wanted to see if I have the willpower to stick to something—with no deviations—for one whole week. And I did! I stuck to it during a week that had two luncheons, a night out for dinner, and a party. I don't even know how much weight, if any, I lost. That was not the point of this experiment. When I went to bed Saturday night I was so proud of myself. I had done what I set out to do. I know I have the willpower to succeed!

SUNDAY, FEBRUARY 25, 1996

A beautiful spring day in Michigan, a rarity for February. The temperature was near 60 degrees, so my husband and I decided to walk the track at our local high school. Tom and I enjoy these outings. In addition to some exercise, we have a chance to talk and catch up with each other. Life has sure changed from our "sit on the couch and watch TV" days.

When we returned home there was a special message on the answering machine. Richard Simmons called me! He really called me! And, he said, he would call back!

MONDAY, FEBRUARY 26, 1996

My editor at Family Circle *called with great news. Richard Simmons has agreed to be my "diet buddy" and to take me to the finish line.*

THURSDAY, FEBRUARY 29, 1996

I did it! I made a major leap this month! *I've had one of the most successful months of my whole programs . . .* No sweets *and no giving in to temptations. I've been completely and absolutely perfect with food (one leg) and exercise (the other leg). I know for sure that I have both feet on the ground and I can make the journey to the end. (Remember my road to success?)*

FRIDAY, MARCH 1, 1996

I am so proud of myself. I am starting this month in such a good place. I have motivated myself and now I have the added help of Richard Simmons. I know that having Richard helping me adds even more responsibility on my part. If he's allowing my name to be connected to his, I am sure he expects results and I have to produce.

There's no turning back and there's no slacking off! The pressure is on! However, this also means that success will be a reality.

MONDAY, MARCH 4, 1996
Richard called to interview me. He asked about each and every member of my family and about their fitness levels. He asked if I was really determined to work with him. He told me he was excited about our working together. I know he will be the demanding coach I now need. I've enjoyed working with Dr. Wagner, but now is the time to move on and "down" with Richard!

TUESDAY, MARCH 12, 1996
I am going to California to spend a few days with Richard. I am so excited and nervous at the same time. I decided to get some clothes for the trip. Guess what! I can now wear most size 20 clothes. This is a big deal considering that I started this program wearing sizes 26 and 28. After looking at new clothes, I decided to wait. Why spend money on clothes when I'll soon be in those smaller teen sizes?

WEDNESDAY, MARCH 13, 1996
Talked to my sisters tonight and told them about the trip. My small-sized sister was very excited for me. However, my sisters with weight problems hardly expressed any interest. I know they are jealous of my success, but they, too, could do what I have done if they only tried. It hasn't been easy, but losing weight and getting fit can be done.

My sisters and others with weight problems think I have been successful because of all the help I've been given—the nutritionist, the health club, exposure in Family Circle. *I can't deny that all these things have contributed to my success. However, I won't let anyone take away the fact that I have worked very hard, day in and day out, to achieve success. There were many, many days when I didn't want to go to the health club to work out, but I went anyway. There have been many, many times when I salivated when looking at tables filled with great food, but I refrained anyway. And there were many nights I went to bed early so I wouldn't be tempted by food. Although I started smoking an occasional cigarette, I am almost cigarette-free again.*

Why do people try to diminish our successes? Why can't they be proud of our achievements?

I guess it is human nature to be jealous of others' good fortune. I know I have been green with envy when others have lost weight. And I've been gleeful when they gained it back! However—and I can honestly say this—I have been supportive of their efforts.

Because of the poor response I have received from my sisters and others with regard to my weight loss, I have learned to keep my mouth shut. (This also helps with the food!) I try not to mention such things as my weight, my clothing size, how much I'm exercising, how much easier my life has become. I try not to say anything about my project.

And I don't have to mention anything. All people have to do is look at me to know that it's working and how hard I'm trying. If they don't say anything, it's okay. I didn't start this program for others, I started it and have been continuing the hard work for myself. I wanted to and have improved my life, and in the process, I've improved my looks. I have given myself something to be proud of. And I am proud of my accomplishments. Self-pride is much more important than the accolades of others.

MONDAY, MARCH 18, 1996
I'm in Beverly Hills, California. I started the day with a mud wrap, a facial, and then had my hair and makeup done. I felt like a virgin

being prepared for sacrifice. This royal treatment was supposed to relax me, but the thought of meeting Richard took the relaxation factor away. I was really nervous.

Arrived at Richard's house for lunch. WOW! He is truly a great host and very warm. He put me at ease immediately. His low-fat lunch was good, too! He sure is observant. He was quick to point out that I am a very fast eater. Jokingly, he named me the winner of the "fastest eater of soup contest." He made his point. I am a very fast eater and I need to slow down to enjoy my food. Also, he served the soup in a teacup, not a soup bowl. He did this to point out that we usually eat too much and by putting it in a teacup, we are getting the correct portion.

Another thing Richard did was to leave the macaroni and cheese main dish in its serving pan on the table after he served each of us the correct portion size. Little did I know this was a test. He watched me after I finished the portion on my plate—a salad plate so I would think I was getting more than I was. "All you kept doing was stare at the rest of the macaroni and cheese," Richard said. He was correct. I kept looking at the food because I wanted more. "And," he added, "If I weren't here you probably would have taken a second helping." Again, Richard was right on! His point in this lesson was that after you dish out the correct portion size, you should remove the remaining food from sight so you won't be tempted.

Richard also commented on my posture. I am a sloucher. He told me to sit up straight . . . to stand tall . . . to always sit and stand like a person who is proud of herself. He said that good posture also helps with breathing.

Throughout lunch I told Richard how proud he was going to be of me, because I was going to reach my goal. He said he was already proud of me; then he told me how good I looked. What a charming man!

Richard spent some private time with me (away from the magazine's camera crew, makeup person, and writer—our meeting would be featured in the October issue) to talk about our journey together. I'm thrilled to have a companion on my road to success. He told me he looked forward to our working together and for me not to be set on losing 70 more pounds. "I don't want you to think you can be the same weight and size you were at twenty-five years of age," he said. I said this was good, because I was really fat at age twenty-five!

Richard told me he would work with me on an exercise program and an eating plan. He ended our time together by stating that we would have a good time working together. I had known this from the moment I met this fun, energetic person. Then we went to his dining room and he gave me a carved egg with a "pixie angel" inside. "This is for you to put someplace in your house so you'll know we're working together!"

That night I had a little more dinner than usual. I was starved. I didn't get to eat very much at lunch. These smaller portions are going to be what leads to success, but they are going to be hard to get used to. My nutritionist has allowed me to eat "unlimited" vegetables and I've filled up on them when I was hungry. Let's see what Richard is going to allow.

When I got back to my room tonight there was a message from Richard on the answering machine. "It was great meeting you and having lunch with you. I look forward to seeing you tomorrow," he said, then added, "Sweet dreams." And that's exactly what I had, sweet dreams.

TUESDAY, MARCH 19, 1996
At 6 P.M. I arrived at Slimmons, Richard's Beverly Hills exercise studio. What a nice welcome he provided. Balloons everywhere and each and every one of his class members made me feel welcome,

beginning with a group "hi" at the curb. I worked out with Richard and, boy, did I feel out of shape. To think that I've been exercising at least six days a week for two years and it was still an effort to keep up with Richard. But I did it! After the class I got one of his famous hugs and kisses and a promise that we'd talk soon.

Returned to my room with another answering machine message from Richard. He told me I did great at the studio and he wished me a "good night."

WEDNESDAY, MARCH 20, 1996

I arrived home at my Beverly Hills with new vigor, determination, and the knowledge that with Richard's help, I will succeed. (Although I had already decided earlier this year that I would not fail!) It's so nice to have someone as dedicated as Richard in my corner.

THURSDAY, MARCH 21, 1996

Richard called today and told me what kind of exercise program he'd like me to follow. Again he proved how observant he is. He told me he had watched me working out at Slimmons and noticed that the upper part of my body was not very strong. He is right! I have been walking six days a week and I work out on the weight machines three days a week. Richard wants me to do more aerobics, to get my arms over my head and to move around more. My new schedule is Monday—walking; Tuesday—aerobics; Wednesday—toning with weights/ weight machines; Thursday—walking; Friday—aerobics; Saturday— toning with weights/weight machines; Sunday—a day off!

SATURDAY, MARCH 30, 1996

Great week . . . my new exercise program is just what I needed. I'm working out less, but I'm working more. I spend less time at the health club, but Richard's plan increases the effectiveness of my workout. He wants me to "mix it up" more. Walking every day does burn calories, but it doesn't provide any variety in my routine. He wanted me to work my upper body more. He added that variety helps keep working out more fun and interesting. Now all I need is my new food plan.

SUNDAY, MARCH 31, 1996

This great month ended with another call from Richard. He told me he needed to see what I've been eating and then he'll develop a food plan for me. He wished me well and told me to keep up the good work. He sang a little bit . . . he talked seriously for a brief time . . . he asked about the family . . . he talked about his mother, Shirley . . . he sounded just like a friend!

TUESDAY APRIL 2—SATURDAY, APRIL 6, 1996

I've been recording every single thing I eat to send to Richard. I think writing down is a good thing. It shows you exactly what you're eating and it helps you concentrate on what you're putting in your mouth. When we don't think about what we're eating, we put a cookie in our mouth here, a few chips there, etc. Another good thing about writing down is that it is a permanent record, and we all want to go on record as being good. So we tend to eat better when we have to write it down.

Richard called this week to ask, "How are you doing?" and, "Can I help you in any way?" He told me how proud he is of me . . . and that I have already made great improvements in my life!

MONDAY, APRIL 8, 1996

I sent Richard a list of everything I ate for the past two weeks so he could assess my dietary needs and develop a food plan for me. My current eating program is based on 1,800 calories a day with lots of carbohydrates and unlimited vegetables.

MONDAY, APRIL 15, 1996

What a taxing day! A friend brought over a lovely cake she made for us. Some people seem to think that because I am dieting my family is being deprived. So there are lots of food gifts for the poor Prysbys. However, I don't think this was the motivation behind this cake. This particular friend is overweight and, through comments, I know she can't stand that I am successfully losing weight. Anyway, I am happy to report that I did not even have a taste of this treat. I did have to go to bed at 9 P.M. to get away from the temptation, but I succeeded. And the next morning I made my family get it out of the house. They did. Thank heaven! If there is one thing I really have it is a tremendous sweet tooth. The family can munch on chips and other such snacks and it doesn't bother me, but bring in a sweet and the temptation is unbearable, especially if it looks and smells good. I try to get the family to have their sweets elsewhere, and most of the time they do.

TUESDAY, APRIL 16, 1996

I started doing Richard Simmons' videotapes at the health club today. I'm doing aerobics twice weekly and the club has given me one of the aerobics rooms with a television to use. I have invited my WOWS members to join me, and today eight of them came for this workout. They loved Richard's "sweating" tapes and I have to admit, he does make working out fun!

WEDNESDAY, APRIL 17, 1996

Got a letter from Richard today. He has analyzed my food sheets. "Some people read tea leaves or palms, I read food sheets," he wrote. And he looked over my exercise program. He said I was doing "terrific" in regards to exercise, but I had to up my workouts. "Right now God gave you seven days. There are no more days off." I guess I can no longer consider Sunday a day of rest!

"Now let's talk food," Richard wrote. "I'm putting diet colas under food because they seem to be a food group for you. You can have two cans a day—the rest water. Why do you get two cups of cereal? I only get one cup." He also suggested that I put some variety in my breakfasts. "Have at least five or six breakfast foods on hand." (He suggested this because I am a creature of habit. I tend to find something I like and I eat it day after day after day.) "How come you get two cups of pasta? I only get one. See what I am trying to get at . . . Your portions are too big!"

I could add more variety for breakfast. I could cut down on my food portions. But cut down on my diet colas! This is going to be a difficult challenge for me. Diet colas carry me through the day, and the caffeine is what keeps me going. What I'm really trying to say is that I am addicted to diet colas . . . big time! But I'll give this a try. I can't go cold turkey. I'll start by reducing my intake one can at a time and work down to two cans a day. Luckily, summer is coming and I usually drink a lot more water in the warm weather.

WEDNESDAY, APRIL 24, 1996

Richard called to outline my new food plan. It's based on 1,500 calories a day. He stressed the point that I must make sure there are three hours between the time I last eat and when I go to bed. He cut my carbohydrates down and limited my veggies. I can live with Rich-

ard's plan. It's sensible and I think it will result in a steadier weight loss.

My Daily Food Plan from Richard

(Approximately 1,500 Calories)

5 proteins
5 starches
2 dairy servings
4 vegetables
4 fruits
4 fats (20 grams)

NOTE: *For selections and serving sizes see Chapter 4, "Food Plan for Life!"*

This plan can be changed to accommodate just about anyone. If you weigh under 150 pounds, you should follow a 1,200-calorie-a-day plan that includes 4 protein, 4 starch, 2 dairy, 3 vegetable, 3 fruit, and 3 fat servings a day.

If you weigh 150–200 pounds, your plan calls for 4 protein, 5 starch, 2 dairy, 4 vegetable, 4 fruit, and 3 fat servings. Those between 200–250 pounds should plan to eat no more than 5 protein, 6 starch, 2 dairy, 5 vegetable, 4 fruit, and 4 fat servings a day.

Sensible eating means having selections from the five food groups. Aside from fats, which should be used sparingly, we need foods from the five food groups for good health. Each group provides specific nutrients our bodies require.

For example, in addition to protein, meat and cheese provide iron, zinc, and some B vitamins. Breads also provide B vitamins, as well as complex carbohydrates and fiber. Dairy products give us calcium (especially important for women), protein, and vitamins A and D. Vegetables and fruits are excellent sources for vitamins A and C, folic acid, and fiber. Some fruits also provide us with potassium.

Chapter 11

From Road "Hog" to Roadrunner!

Toot! Toot! Just like the cartoon roadrunner seen speeding down desert roads, I'm moving more quickly toward my goal, thanks to Richard and the new food plan he developed for me.

Richard is a great motivator. He expects me to succeed and to stay on track—more specifically, on the road to good health and fitness. And he has a way about him that makes me want to do just what he expects, what he knows will work. In his own fun way and with deep concern and empathy, Richard gently pushes me and makes me want to work harder. He's a good trainer who is full of kind words. However, I know he expects me to do what needs to be done.

Also, I like my new food plan. It's easy to follow and allows choices. Because of it, I am eating smaller portions and less bread. I don't feel stuffed after I eat. I'm not hungry, just not so full. I like this feeling.

Another good thing about the food plan, and, more important, Richard's philosophy, is that, on occasion, I can "save up" foods and eat them at the many functions my husband and I (we're social animals) attend. (This wasn't encouraged under my previous food plan and I often felt deprived at luncheons, dinners, and parties.)

Richard's food plan and the "save up" policy fit my lifestyle. And, because of this, I'm having no trouble sticking to healthy, sensible eating.

WEDNESDAY, MAY 1, 1996

I am developing new habits and strategies that are helping me. Here's one that I use. When I have a craving for something bad, after I get it out of the refrigerator or cupboard I set it down on the counter and leave the room. I go into the living room, which has floor to ceiling mirrors, look at my reflection, and then have a talk with myself about eating the forbidden food. If, after a few minutes, I still want to eat the food, I eat it. However, most times I don't! If I'm not at home when these cravings hit, I still have a talk with myself, only it's in my head. I have found that my conscious mind is quite smart and I don't unconsciously put food in my mouth anymore!

EXCERPT FROM LETTER TO RICHARD SIMMONS, MAY 13, 1996

In our short relationship, you've managed to help me achieve some wonderful successes. I'm now exercising seven days a week, and, on nice days, I even do double duty by walking the track near my home. This is in addition to my regular exercise program. Either my husband or one of the children joins me on the track. I've discovered the family that walks together, talks together!

Also, and this is a "biggie," I am reducing my diet colas. It's been difficult, but I'm doing it!

EXCERPT FROM LETTER FROM RICHARD SIMMONS,
MAY 19, 1996

You really are exercising. Wait, I think you are doing more than me!

FRIDAY, MAY 24, 1996

Got on the scale today. I weigh 222! I know why I am losing weight again. Richard has me on the right amount of calories and a nice mix of exercise. If I had continued with my former food plan, I'm not sure I would ever have reached my goal. It was healthy food, but too much!

TUESDAY, MAY 28–SUNDAY, JUNE 2, 1996

Today begins a very big challenge. I am going on a six-day trip to the World Finals for Odyssey of the Mind in Ames, Iowa. Each year when I go to this competition I really blow it! This year I vowed it would be different. I would be perfect!

On the ten-hour trip to Ames, my two traveling companions and I made various stops including fast-food restaurants and gas stations. There were lots of food temptations, but I didn't give in to one, not one.

The whole time I was in Ames I followed my food plan perfectly. My crowning achievement was at the officials party Saturday night. This gigantic party had every kind of food imaginable, including baby back ribs (my favorite), cheesecakes and pastries (also my downfall), and appetizers galore. I was tempted so much that three times I stood in line for food. Three times I got to the head of the line, but left and returned to the table minus food. The only thing I ate that evening was a handful of popcorn, and a small handful at that! I really didn't want anything else, even though I had "saved up" for the party.

I ended this trip to Iowa very, very proud of myself. I had control over food, it didn't have control over me. I am doing it . . . and it no longer is too difficult. It has been a very long time since I goofed!

Doing well is a great motivator. One good meal leads to the next good meal; one good day encourages the next good day. When these good days extend to a week or more, doing well no longer is a goal, but a necessity. Who wants to undo everything they've done? I know I don't. I want the cycle to continue and, because of this, I refuse to take even a bite of anything not listed on my food plan.

I am very fortunate to have inspiration in my own home, someone who has shown me the benefits of motivation. It's my daughter Libby.

For a number of years Libby has achieved straight As on her report card, and these grades have been earned in the more difficult honors classes. Libby is the type of person who does what she has to do, and then some. She doesn't do the work to get As. She just does the work the very best she can, and because of this, she gets the top grades.

Libby's fine example has inspired me in my weight-loss efforts. I now do what I have to do, the best I can, and I'm getting good grades, top grades. And I want to maintain my perfect record!

SATURDAY, JUNE 8, 1996
Since spring arrived I have been walking the track every night after dinner. I hate the time after dinner and until it gets dark. To me, it's a lost time. Too early to settle in to watch television and too late to start a big project. So I walk the track. I do at least two miles, sometimes three. This is in addition to my daily workouts at the health club.

I love walking the track. I'm outside in the fresh air and, unlike when I walk on a treadmill, I swing my arms. It's great exercise and my body feels wonderful when I go to bed. No longer do I have heartburn at night. These walks help me digest my dinner.

SUNDAY, JUNE 9, 1996

Andy's seventeenth birthday and I didn't have a piece of his cake. Refraining from sweets and continuing my quest for good health are the best presents I can give any of my kids.

EXCERPT FROM LETTER TO RICHARD SIMMONS,
JUNE 12, 1996

I figured out why everything is "working" with you. I liken myself to an athlete, and you are my coach. To be a really good athlete I need a goal, some skill, desire, and an excellent coach who can help me develop my skills and keep me focused. Also, to be a successful athlete I need to practice, practice, practice.

I have the goal—to lose weight and be fit and healthy; the skill— I am lucky God blessed me with a good brain to know what I should and shouldn't do to reach my goal; the desire—it continues to be strong and, because of this, I practice, practice, practice (eat right and exercise). And I have an excellent coach.

Well, Coach Richard, you have given me the tools (food plan and exercise program). And, like a good coach, you also know your stuff. Finally, the most important thing you have given me, Coach, is your belief in me.

I'm in training to be the best I can be. Not only do I want to be proud of myself, I want you to be proud of me. That's what happens when an athlete admires and trusts her coach!

FRIDAY, JUNE 28, 1996
I made a big mistake tonight and boy did I pay for it! At midnight my son decided to go on a Taco Bell run. It's been months since I've had Mexican food so I asked him to bring me one taco, just one taco. I ate it and then spent the night in tremendous pain. I had heartburn so bad that I felt I was dying—all from one taco. Never, never again!

EXCERPT FROM LETTER FROM RICHARD SIMMONS, JUNE 30, 1996
Your food sheets were so heavenly they floated out of the envelope. Do you own stock in diet colas? These are filled with so much sodium, Sandy.

Food sheets and writing down what I eat. I guess I can't get away from this task. And there's a good reason for it. According to experts, successful weight loss results when you are aware of what you eat. Also, Richard checks these weekly food sheets (that's how he knows about my continued diet cola addiction) and makes suggestions and recommendations.

Although it would be nice, you don't need an expert, a Richard, to check your food sheets. And you don't need food sheets per se. You can use a notebook, a piece of paper, a computer, just about anything. What you do need is to write down what you eat. (I believe you need to go a step further. You should also write down the night before what foods you plan to eat the next day. You need to plan!)

In addition to keeping a log of what you eat and how much water you drink (also important), you should jot down what exercises you participate in daily. This record, if you are honest in your entries, will help you determine where and when difficulties occur, and, more important, where changes are needed. You can be your own expert. You can make the adjustments needed for success. But you have to know where you're at in order to direct your journey to fitness and good health.

EXCERPT FROM LETTER TO RICHARD SIMMONS,
JULY 10, 1996

I officially reached my 100-pound weight loss and I did it at a very special time—the Fourth of July weekend! Now I have independence from fat! And you thought all those fireworks across America were for something else!!!

SATURDAY, JULY 13, 1996

I went shopping today and decided I deserved a treat. After all, I have been so good for so long. I picked ice cream as the lucky winner. I went to the freezers to select my treat. I walked back and forth checking each and every carton and container. I checked the fat content, the calories, the ingredients, the price. I wanted the very best and the most luscious. If I was going to cheat, it was going to be a big cheat. For half an hour I checked and rechecked. I was there for so long that one of the employees asked if I needed help. I went back and forth from brand to brand. Back and forth. I then made a decision. I didn't need a treat. My treat is how wonderful I look and feel! I didn't need ice cream!

FRIDAY, JULY 26, 1996

Walking the track is great, but it's getting too congested. So many people have seen me on my daily track walks (the track is next to a busy main street and my white hair is very noticeable) that they have showed up to walk with me. One night this week there were six friends. I don't like this. My track walking is not a social outing, it's exercise and my little solace from everyday aggravations. Now I change the time I walk so no one knows my pattern. Sometimes I go to another track at another school. I am a serious walker, while my friends consider walking the track "social exercise." I now do a fifteen-minute mile and few can keep up with me.

SUNDAY, JULY 28, 1996

Today Tom and I went sailing. I haven't done this for years because it was always so hard to get in and out of the boat and to move around on it. However, today was different! I was able, on my own, to climb up into the boat and climb back out of it. I cannot believe my newfound flexibility. It comes not only from the weight loss, but also from the daily exercise. Our friends were so happy we joined them. They have asked us before and I always declined. Now I don't have to make up excuses . . . I am a sailor again!

THURSDAY, AUGUST 1, 1996

Now that I am getting totally fit, I've decided to add a new challenge on the first of every month, or at least something different. Today I decided to see if I could walk five miles in one hour. That's a twelve-minute mile. And you know what, I did it! It practically killed me, but I did it.

FRIDAY, AUGUST 2–SUNDAY, AUGUST 4, 1996

One of those amazing weekends consisting of a number of social gatherings, all revolving around food. However, unlike the past, I can control my food in these situations and eat healthy. And, not only that, I can enjoy the occasion without feeling deprived. Salads are good . . . fresh fruit is good . . . there are things to eat at social gatherings.

FRIDAY, AUGUST 30–SATURDAY, AUGUST 31, 1996

A holiday weekend, but I'm not afraid. I now know how to handle those special times that used to give me an excuse for cheating. Parties and barbecues fill this weekend, but I don't have to worry. Instead I look forward to being with friends and meeting new people. I love going out now. I'm just a normal-sized person with maybe a little more weight to lose. I'm not obese anymore. I now have confidence in the way I look.

Now I have lots and lots of loose clothes. It's great to "swim" in clothes. It's great when hose stay up and don't ramble down rolls and rolls of fat and hug the knees. It's nice when buttons don't pop open on the front of blouses. It's wonderful when tops don't hug my bosom so tightly that they reduce my bust size by inches and transform me into a streetwalker. It's gratifying that my tummy is so flat now that I no longer look twelve months pregnant.

I'm ending this month feeling good and doing great. This is the best way to enjoy life!

SUNDAY, SEPTEMBER 1, 1996

It's the first of the month and time for a new challenge. I can't believe what I did today!

It was a beautiful fall day. All the kids were gone from the house. Tom was outside cutting the grass. We were home alone! I climbed into the shower and after using fragrant bath oil I went nude out to our patio. (It's almost a private patio, but not quite.) I called to Tom. It took a while for him to respond because of the noise of the lawn mower. (Hopefully, none of the neighbors witnessed this scene!) When he finally turned his head and saw me, his eyes got big and a smile came to his face. I told him to come now. He did! And we did!

This was the first time in years that I had initiated sex. I had become disgusted with my body and didn't feel comfortable coming on to Tom. Now I feel better about my body; I feel like an attractive woman. I flirt with Tom more . . . I let him touch me more. However, it took today and my nude appearance before him to make me feel like a woman. And, boy, did Tom appreciate it. He said he could hardly wait to see what I was going to do on October 1, our wedding anniversary.

EXCERPT FROM LETTER FROM RICHARD SIMMONS,
SEPTEMBER 2, 1996

Just finished looking at your food sheets. Gosh, you love hamburgers. You love meat. You love pizza. You are my kind of girl! Cut down your red meat intake. A couple nights a week make a salad, and make it interesting, my sweet kissing cousin.

SATURDAY, SEPTEMBER 7, 1996

Libby and I met Richard in Toledo, where he was giving a talk as part of that city's Women's Health Day. Richard treated us like royalty. We met him at his suite for a private visit (Libby said it was like having an audience with the Pope), and then we went by limo with him to his talk. (He's great onstage.) He introduced us to the fifteen hundred audience members. Afterward, many attendees came up to me and asked to take my picture and for an autograph. Our day ended with Richard and the limo taking us back to our car and Richard giving me a dozen red roses. What a man!

EXCERPT FROM LETTER TO RICHARD SIMMONS,
SEPTEMBER 9, 1996.

How lucky I was the day you entered my life. Losing weight has nothing to do with this feeling. Meeting a person like you, someone so truly unselfish and giving, is what has enhanced my life. I have become a better person through your example. I no longer think of you as just that "always on, always funny, always motivational diet guru." To me you are one of life's special people . . . one of God's angels sporting sequins and an Afro.

SUNDAY, SEPTEMBER 15, 1996
Richard called today to ask me to go to Philly and be on the QVC shopping network with him. He said he wants to keep me motivated.

MONDAY, SEPTEMBER 16–FRIDAY, SEPTEMBER 20, 1996
I shopped this week for a few new clothes for the QVC appearances. I went to my regular plus-size shops and discovered an amazing thing. I have "undergrown" plus sizes. I was excited, but a little depressed, too. For years I knew where to shop and what to buy. Now I didn't even know what size (it's Misses large, I learned) or what style to buy. I have been wearing "cover-up" clothes forever . . . now what!

MONDAY, SEPTEMBER 23, 1996
The new session of WOWS began today and sixteen women signed up. This class has really grown. More than seventy women have gone through it and are now regular members of the health club. These are women who didn't exercise on a regular basis and would never have considered a health club setting if it weren't for WOWS. This success makes me feel good, because I know I am helping a whole bunch of women get fit. I'm doing good at the same time I'm achieving my goals.

I weighed in at 195 pounds today!!! Based on my high of 325 pounds this means I am down 130 pounds. (It was 115 pounds down from my Family Circle start.) That's a person I've lost!

WEDNESDAY, SEPTEMBER 25–FRIDAY,
SEPTEMBER 27, 1996

In Philly doing QVC show. I had great fun with Richard, but, then again, who wouldn't! On the last show Richard gave me a string of 130 pearls to mark each pound I've lost. What a surprise and what a nice ending to an exciting experience. Each time I talk to Richard or see him, I gain more respect for him.

SATURDAY, SEPTEMBER 28, 1996

I wore the pearls Richard gave me to a wedding tonight. An astonishing thing happened. Whenever I got near fattening food, the pearls started to choke me. When I moved away from these bad foods, the necklace lessened its grip. How does Richard do this?????

(Of course, this really didn't happen! However, the pearls did serve as a reminder of the 130 pounds I've lost, so, in a way, they worked. They kept me away from the unhealthy offerings.)

TUESDAY, OCTOBER 1, 1996

My nineteenth wedding anniversary and time for my first-of-the-month challenge. Tom got what he wanted (me, too), and I added a strenuous new exercise—the StairMaster machine—to my program.

SUNDAY, OCTOBER 20, 1996

While I was at the checkout counter at the grocery store I saw two magazines with miracle diets. I bought them. I still have a problem with wanting to go fast and do a diet that gets instant results. I know better! And I know that what I am doing—following a good food plan for life—is the right way to achieve results. However, I guess old habits are hard to lose!

WEDNESDAY, OCTOBER 23, 1996

Richard was in town today on his book tour and I was able to spend some time with him. More important, Tom, Andy, and Emily got to meet "the other man" in my life. (Libby had this chance in Toledo.) The whole family is impressed with this energetic weight-loss wonder!

SUNDAY, NOVEMBER 3, 1996

My fifty-second birthday. Who would have guessed that I would be so fit on this birthday considering where I was a few years ago? I don't feel fifty-two (whatever that's supposed to feel like) . . . I feel better than I did when I was in my thirties. I feel young and my body acts as if it's young!

As a birthday treat to myself I decided to have an absolutely perfect week on the food plan. No straying. Everything I put into my mouth will be weighed and measured. Sometimes I get lazy with weighing and measuring. After all, I figure, I've been on this program so long I can "eyeball" portions. Wrong! It's amazing how a cup can creep up to almost two cups and 4 ounces can really be 7 ounces. I have to measure and weigh more frequently to be successful.

I'm now down to 183—imagine, 183 pounds. Some people would be dismayed with this number. I love it!

MONDAY, NOVEMBER 18, 1996

Every Monday I give a thirty-minute motivational talk for the women in my WOWS class. This session has sixteen members. Some—those who have made a real commitment to themselves—are doing well. The others are using the class as a social outing and making excuses for why they are not losing weight. At least all of

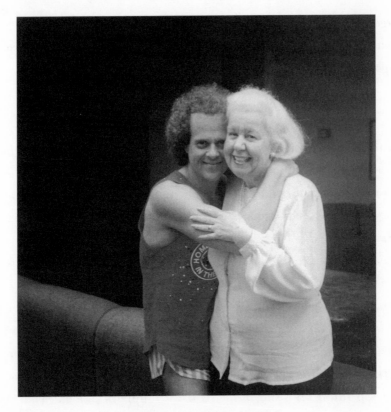

Getting up close with Richard.

them are exercising four times a week, so they are making a difference in their lives.

My topic today was "Getting Through the Holidays Successfully." I love giving these talks because they serve as reminders to
myself of what I have to do to be successful. I plan to have a better
holiday season this year, even with all the parties. I plan to eat
healthy—no exceptions. I told my class and myself that planning is
the only way to handle the holidays. Having the refrigerator stocked
with good foods—make that healthy foods—will help decrease the

urge to eat all the junk that comes into our homes at this time of year. Having a plan is the only way to be successful. You can't reach a goal without a plan.

THANKSGIVING 1996

With all my good intentions I never thought I would blow the first event of the holiday season. However, thanks to my sister-in-law and my lack of planning, I did! Tom, the kids, and I went to Tom's sister's cottage for the Thanksgiving weekend. She assured me that we didn't need to bring any food, everything was taken care of. She has always been enthusiastic about my weight-loss program, so I assumed that she would have lots of healthy foods for me. Wrong! Just about every-thing was bad. High-fat foods and snacks. For breakfast she had egg dishes (they did taste good) and coffee cake. For Thanksgiving dinner she had a salad that probably had more fat grams than the whole turkey itself. And all the vegetables were trapped in cream sauces. Do you think my sister-in-law is a true supporter? I ate what was served, but sparingly, but still I ate badly. So much so that I was up all night with heartburn. Also, I had planned to walk for exercise. No way. The cottage is on a bluff in a very hilly area. The ground was covered with snow and ice. There was nowhere to walk. Get me home! I need my healthy food and exercise!

EXCERPT FROM LETTER TO RICHARD SIMMONS, DECEMBER 2, 1996

I am planning to do well during the holiday season (although I goofed on Thanksgiving). This year I have a plan—and the plan is to be successful. I will stay away from the food tables, carry pretzels and a small bag of carrots to the parties. More important, I will go to each and every event with the resolve to do good. (I'll use your little tip of looking in the mirror before leaving home and commending myself on how far I've come! This should keep me from blowing it!)

Every time I write to Richard, or hear from him via letter or telephone call, I think about all he has done for me. He's helped me with the food; he's encouraged the exercise. However, his greatest contribution to my success is his concern. He cares about me. He cares about my family. I consider him a friend, a rare friend who gives of himself without expecting any reward except my success.

I wanted to give something to Richard, especially during this season of giving. I was stymied. What could I give to a man who probably has everything he needs? Besides, financially there was nothing I could afford that would come close to the great "wealth" he has given me.

An idea came to mind. I went to the grocery store and purchased bottles of Cheer (laundry soap) and Joy (dish soap). I asked a friend of mine to take a picture of me, dressed in an apron and wearing my pearls (and other clothes, too) and holding the two soaps. With this picture for Richard, I sent the following tale:

A GOODBYE TO FAT TAIL (OOPS! MAKE THAT TALE!)
Once upon a time in the faraway village of Beverly Hills, in the land of Michigan, there lived a woman known throughout the realm for her mirth and large girth and her white hair. The mother of three and the wife of one, this woman was not totally happy. Oh sure, her family was wonderful, her friends numerous and true, but there was something missing. There was little Joy and Cheer in her life, for her large girth thwarted her from partaking in many of the universe's offerings.

One day, in a distant part of the kingdom, a Prince of a Fellow—

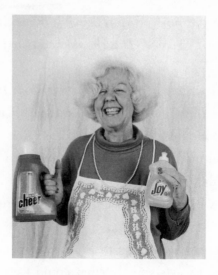

Joy and Cheer. MAUREEN ELECTA MONTE

one known far and wide for his Joy and Cheer—heard of the plight of the woman known for her mirth and girth and her white hair. This prince, with trademark hair of his own, unselfishly hurried to rescue this dame in distress (which was not unusual, for this was the lifelong quest of this noble man among men). His new mission was to instill in this dame with the mirth and girth lots of Joy and Cheer and Good Fitness, too!

This pleasant prince would personally prevail to help the distressed dame say goodbye to fat!

So the handsome and dashing prince, armed with wisdom (and a multitude of fitness products), lent an ear, shared his time, and offered his concern for the woman from afar. He assured the woman with the white hair that her girth—with effort—would go, and her mirth—with constant replenishment—would increase. But the most amazing gift he offered—if the dame dare do the deed—was a Healthy Lifestyle of good nutrition and exercise.

An alliance was formed, the goal was set, and the pleasing prince and the delighted dame went forth to success.

Much girth has been lost, with more to go, and Joy and Cheer are now filling the heart and hearth of the now dazzling dame.

Now the prince, being a generous sovereign, bestowed upon this dame a most luminous and long string of pearls as a reward for saying goodbye to fat. This awesome award has transformed the woman with less girth and more mirth—you know, the delighted dame with white hair—into something most unusual. Armed with her Joy and Cheer, and now sporting her pearls, this once distressed dame is known far and wide as the "MaDonna Reed-like of Beverly Hills!" (In olden times, with her great girth and her lack of pearls, she was unable to clean up her act! No problem now!)

Her family is ecstatic, her friends are, too, and all in her kingdom thank Prince Richard for being so true.

DECEMBER 31, 1996

New Year's Eve. A trip to the scales made me really feel good. I just nudged into the 170s—at 179 pounds. I made my year-end goal! What a nice way to start 1997!

Chapter 12

Down, Down, Down!

I'm going down the road, down the scale, and down the dress sizes. At the same time, my self-esteem is going up!

Self-esteem. Four years ago my self-esteem was really suffering. How could it not? My twelve-year-old daughter was shaving my legs. (I couldn't reach down to perform this basic female task.) My ten-year-old daughter was tying my shoelaces before she left for school. (I couldn't reach down to my feet.) My fourteen-year-old son went grocery shopping with me to get items on the lower shelves. (No way could I bend down.) Everything in my life at that time seemed to be "down," especially my self-esteem. My excess weight got in the way of just about everything.

My husband and the kids handled many of the household tasks. I didn't have the energy or the agility to do much around the house. I was the homemaker, but it took my family to make the home livable.

Four years ago I felt both blessed and depressed when my loved ones readily, without complaint, completed necessary chores. While my excess weight was overworking my heart and other organs, it was also overworking my family. I hated each and every time I had to request help from my family. I felt like a failure—an awful wife and mother!

TUESDAY, JANUARY 7, 1997

I didn't think I would ever say this, but "doing housework is a joy!" I like having a clean house and now I have one. It's not perfect, but it's clean. And I'm the one doing most of the cleaning. I'm giving Tom and the kids a break. They've done more than their share over the years. Besides, I have so much energy now that I can do the work myself.

SATURDAY, JANUARY 11, 1997

When I bought new panty hose today I realized I now fit into the regular sizes. I'm no queen now, just one of the regulars!

I love being in regular sizes. I can shop just about anywhere for clothes and now I don't have to pay extra. (When you place catalog orders, the plus sizes always run about five dollars more than the regular sizes. I guess it's because of the extra material needed for the garment. What I don't understand is why petites aren't $5 less! Oh well, I'll never have to worry about being petite. I'm too tall!)

FRIDAY, JANUARY 17, 1997

Richard called tonight. He said he's very proud of how well I'm doing. He is definitely a super uplift. It's nice having him to report to. He stressed my need to drink more water (and fewer diet colas).

MONDAY, JANUARY 20, 1997

Today I added bicycling to my exercise program. I am really motivated when it comes to exercise. I just like the way my body feels when I finish my workout. And I like the way my body works when I am working out. It feels like a well-running machine!

While many of my friends have intimated that I have become an exercise addict, this is far from true. I have yet to learn to love exercise; I have yet to become obsessed with it. I limit my workouts to approximately one and a half hours a day, seven days a week. Walking, bicycling, and working a few minutes on my abs are the foundation of my workout. Then I add weight training and toning three days a week and aerobics (doing a Richard Simmons video, water aerobics, or cardioboxing) twice a week. Sometimes I do a little extra walking or bicycling if one of the kids or my husband wants to work out in the evening. And, if the weather is good, there is rarely a time when my husband and I don't go for a walk—not a leisurely stroll but a walk at a fast cardiovascular pace.

Okay! Okay! I know what you're saying. You just don't have the time for this much exercise. Well, folks, neither do I. But I do it, and it's made all the difference.

This may seem like a lot of exercise, but it isn't. It's just a good varied program. Many times I exercise with friends (it's better than going to lunch) or with family members. However, my companions have to keep up with my fast pace. It's better than wasting time watching TV and the rewards have been great. It has not only enabled me to lose weight, but I have more flexibility than I have ever had, including when I was in my teens and twenties. I can't believe how good my body feels and how well it performs! And I have *energy*. Boy, do I have energy! I accomplish more than I ever did, even with a demanding schedule. Remember, I have three very active and involved teenagers and a husband who needs a little attention once in a while! Also, I have a freelance writing business; I teach six WOWS classes a week; I teach storytelling and creative writing classes to elementary school students; and I am one of our community's most active volunteers. I'm in my fifties but I can do all this because *I take time each day for exercise!*

FRIDAY, JANUARY 24, 1997

One major improvement in my life is that I rarely overindulge in foods—especially fatty foods, my previous favorites. Slow but sure has been the best way to go. I have learned so much and I can truly say that I have developed a healthy lifestyle—one I can and will follow for life. My body has become accustomed to healthy foods and it doesn't like high-fat ones (gas, heartburn, diarrhea).

FRIDAY, JANUARY 31, 1997

I ended the month at 175 pounds. I can't believe this! I'm also wearing size 14 (mostly) and size 16 (rarely) clothes.

SATURDAY, FEBRUARY 1, 1997

I am so agile. Today I picked up a penny from the ground. I didn't even give it a second thought when I bent down to retrieve it. A few years ago I would never have bent down to pick up a coin. Not even a quarter. That's because I couldn't do it. I was too fat. When I was a child my mother told me that finding a penny was lucky. It meant, according to her, a wish would come true! I now think of all those wishes that went unfulfilled because I left pennies on the ground. I'm lucky now!

FRIDAY, FEBRUARY 14, 1997

Valentine's Day. My husband gave me a new wedding band (he said he'd marry me again) because my other ring kept falling off. The new ring is a size 6 . . . this compared to the size 10 I wore when I was 300-plus pounds. Also, I finally got some new underpants.

They're size 8 and they're a little big. These replace the stretched-out ones that were falling off me. No wonder. My old ones stretched from size 11 to size 14.

Smaller sizes and looking good! These are such grand benefits of losing weight. Although I didn't begin this weight-loss program to look good, I like looking good!

The main motivation for this program was to get fit and healthy and, if possible, extend my life. I didn't want to die prematurely and leave Tom to finish the task of raising our three children alone. Of all people, Tom does not need to lose me, especially when I can do something to improve my health.

When I met my husband he was a single father of an eighteen-month-old daughter. His wife had died six months earlier. She had experienced postpartum depression after the birth of their daughter. This condition soon progressed into the more severe form, postpartum psychosis. For almost a year, as his wife battled her illness both in and out of hospitals, Tom had the responsibility of holding down his job, assisting his wife, and caring for baby Laura. It was a very difficult year, which ended a few days before Laura's first birthday. His wife committed suicide.

Tom, armed with great faith in God's goodness, chose to put this tragedy in the past and give Laura a good life. He, Laura, and then, luckily, I, were inseparable. However, tragedy struck again. In February 1977, Tom's cherished two-year-old daughter died of Reye's syndrome, a rare but often deadly disease.

My husband had lost so much in his life. He didn't need to lose me, too. I had and have a special responsibility to do everything to keep myself healthy and fit.

SATURDAY, FEBRUARY 22, 1997

I needed to borrow my daughter's slip tonight. (Mine slipped right down over my hips.) I can't believe I am borrowing my daughters' clothes. (Neither can they!)

MONDAY, MARCH 31, 1997

I'm down to 165 pounds. The road ahead is getting short and I still have the motivation and energy—in fact, even more than when I started—to complete the journey. How can this be? Wasn't I supposed to give up long ago? I always did before. What's made the difference this time? Of all the things that have been instrumental in my success, there are four that, I believe, are the answer—God's help, family support, a realistic and livable food plan, and exercise.

How did I, and do I, stay so committed to exercise? I'm asked this several times a week by those who think what I'm doing is almost unnatural. (What is unnatural is not moving our limbs. If God wanted us to stay stationary, He wouldn't have given us joints!)

The reason I continue to exercise on a regular basis (besides the fact that my body feels so good when I'm done) is how I view this activity. I consider exercise my part-time job. And, just like a job, if I don't do it I'll get fired (a very negative thing). Also, because it's a job, I never, ever make appointments with doctors or dentists or plan other activities during work hours. Sure, occasional emergencies can change the schedule, but these are rare.

Your "part-time job" may be during the morning hours (some say this is best: you get it over with and out of the way) or you may "work" (out) at night. I'm a 1–3 P.M. worker. (I can be home by the time the kids get home from school.)

THURSDAY, APRIL 10, 1997

Richard continues to call, write, and offer support. He fears that at the rate I'm going, I'll weigh less than he does. I don't care about weight. I just want to have a quarter of the energy he has. Fat chance! (There's that word "fat" again!)

TUESDAY, APRIL 15, 1997

Today wasn't a "taxing" day. For the first time in our married life, I filed our income taxes long before they were due. (Maybe being on track in one segment of my life is affecting the other areas!) I was very proud of myself for being so organized. I decided to reward myself with a treat. No! Not food! Those days are gone! I would take my measurements. This would be my treat. I hadn't done this in over three years. It was time.

	9/1993	4/1997
bust	54″	40″
waist	50″	34″
hips	57½″	41″
upper arm (l)	16″	12″
upper arm (r)	17″	12″
calves	20″	15″

I can't believe it. I've lost 65½ inches. I never realized how well I was doing. Now I know why my clothes are falling off me!

WEDNESDAY, APRIL 23, 1997

A few more benefits of weight loss. I can now sleep on my stomach. It was painful to sleep in this position when my breasts and midriff were so large. Now I'm comfortable. Also, and this is exciting, I can wrap a bath towel (notice I said "towel," not the large bath "sheet") around my body. I always thought this looked sexy on actresses in movies. Now I'm the sexy one! I'm the star!

SATURDAY, MAY 3, 1997
My victorious return to Washington! Four years ago, a family trip to our nation's capital caused me extreme distress. This trip is a source of joy! Emily is receiving an award for being Michigan's top middle school volunteer from Prudential and the National Association of Secondary School Principals. What an honor! And I get to go with her to the festivities. It involves lots of tours; lots of walking. I'm ready. I'm so slender now and so physically fit that I can enjoy this adventure.

While I was on this trip I was reminded of my early days and the importance I placed, even as a young child, on having a seat no matter where I was. To make sure that I always had a place to sit, I would drag, and later carry, my rocking chair to friends' houses when I went out to play. While the other kids ran around I would happily sit and rock in my chair. I did this so often that the seat's black luster finish soon wore down to the wood. The runners also took a beating from constant transportation.

Many times while in Washington, I chose not to sit, even when I had the opportunity. Now I like to stand . . . and this makes me feel I have an advantage over others. Standing versus sitting also makes me feel young. Only old people (and certain little girls) need to sit. This I don't need. I can stand up for myself now!

TUESDAY, MAY 6, 1997
What a wondrous trip. And what wondrous food! I ate it all, but only small amounts of each offering. I didn't deprive myself, but I also didn't go overboard. I now eat only when I am hungry and only until

I'm full. I even leave food on my plate. I have finally given up my membership in the Clean Plate Club.

FRIDAY, MAY 9, 1997

I gained a few pounds on my four-day sojourn, but they are already gone. Most have heard "fast off, fast on." This is the curse of diets. Take off pounds fast and they come back just as fast. I've turned this around. I've done "fast on, fast off." This is the blessing of a healthy food plan and a slow but sure weight loss!

SUNDAY, MAY 18, 1997

Another trip and another challenge. Let's see if I can handle the food and exercise. I leave tomorrow for five days in New York. Family Circle is planning a makeover, clothes shopping, a fashion shoot (yep! a real NYC fashion shoot), and some time and pictures with Richard Simmons in Central Park. I'm very excited, but nervous, too! Have I lost enough weight for the editors of Family Circle? The scales says I have—I'm now 154 pounds—but do I really look like it?

MONDAY, MAY 19, 1997

Hurray! I discovered a food establishment specializing in salads—all kinds of healthy salads—around the corner from my hotel. Also, my hotel has a great gym with all the equipment I need. I'm going to do just great on this trip. Also—and this is the best part—my Family Circle editors think I look fantastic! They are extremely proud of me. I guess I have "done good"!

TUESDAY, MAY 20, 1997

I walked to and from the hair salon (a total of six miles). I could have taken a taxi, but I chose to walk (that's what I do now). And a light New York rainfall didn't stop me. At the salon I got a new perky

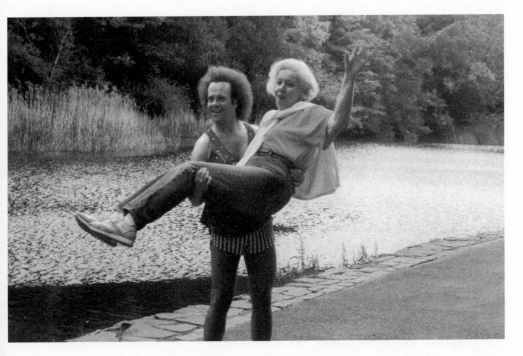

In Central Park with Richard. Being 155 pounds is very uplifting.

hairdo and a color wash—my white hair has an ash-blond tone to it
now. And I got a full body massage. The massage therapist gave me a
choice. I could keep my underwear on, or I could go nude with a
towel over me. I did it! I went nude! I have become comfortable
enough with my body that I can take all my clothes off! What freedom!

WEDNESDAY, MAY 21, 1997
*Size 12! That's the size clothes I wear. What a shock! It took a
shopping trip in New York to discover my new size. Who would have
guessed! And I got my first pair of jeans in years—designer jeans,
thank you!*

THURSDAY, MAY 22, 1997

Richard Simmons picked me up in Central Park. Not that kind of pickup! He literally picked me up in his arms and held me. And he didn't get a hernia for his efforts!

It's been a very long time since a man has picked me up. My husband did carry me over the threshold on our wedding day almost twenty years ago, but I was 163 pounds then and that number soon ballooned.

The last time I was lifted by the opposite sex was seven years ago, and it took not one but two men to do the job. It happened one evening when I experienced severe chest pains. They got so bad my husband called EMS. The two technicians who arrived to help decided I needed to be transported to the hospital. They had great difficulty lifting me from my bed to the gurney, and again lifting the gurney into the ambulance. Even in severe pain, I could see the men straining and hear the groans caused by my excess weight. I was more than embarrassed. I was mortified. Also I was worried that it had finally happened. I was sure that my unhealthy lifestyle had finally resulted in a heart attack. I left the house with my three babies in tears and the fear that I would never see them again.

I spent three days in the hospital's cardiac care unit. All around me were machines and next to me was an elderly roommate near death. It was a sobering experience. I was greatly relieved when the final diagnosis was made: heartburn. My unhealthy eating habits, and probably the more than fifty cigarettes I smoked a day, had put me in the hospital.

Now wouldn't you think that this major scare would change my life, or, at the very least, change my diet? It didn't. I would experience several more bouts with heartburn over the years before I did something "cool" for my heart!

FRIDAY, MAY 23, 1997

I felt elegant today modeling my new clothes for the camera. (Family Circle is planning to use these pictures for its September issue to announce my success.) All the clothes are in neutral tones and are fitted. What a change from my fat days. Formerly, I chose to wear not only big, body-covering clothes, but bright—the brighter the better— garments. I didn't want to hide in black and other dark colors, a common practice among overweight individuals. (Dark colors are supposed to make the wearer look slimmer. At 325 pounds, nothing made me look slim!) I wore bright colors in order to present myself as an optimistic, fun-loving person. I draped myself in pinks (mostly fuchsia), blues (mostly turquoise), purples, and reds. I was a stand-out!

Now I don't need colors to make a statement. With the weight loss has come a quiet confidence in how I look. I like the elegance of neutrals. I like the sophistication of black and navy. I don't need dark colors to hide my weight. I now use them to enhance my figure. A figure! That's what I now have!

SUNDAY, JUNE 1, 1997

Ever since my children began playing sports I was restricted to the bottom bleachers. I couldn't climb to the top where everybody else sat. Many times I felt left out. My weight kept me from joining the other parents and prevented me from getting a good view of the action on the playing field.

Today I went to Emily's soccer game and I climbed up and sat on the very top bleacher with the other parents. I was just one of the group. And I had a perfect view of Emily's game-winning goal! It's great being on top!

SUNDAY, JUNE 8, 1997

Lots of pictures today as we celebrated the high school graduation and eighteenth birthday of our Andrew. I didn't shy away from the camera. I was very proud to stand next to my handsome son and the rest of the family for these memorable pictures. There are too few photos of me with my children over the years. I didn't want a permanent record of my excessive weight. What a loss!

SATURDAY, JUNE 14, 1997

I did something terrible today, something I vowed I would never do. I picked on both of my daughters about their weight.

The family attended a graduation party for a friend. When the girls returned from the buffet table with plates heaped with food I said, "Do you need all that?" Both girls—rightly—became very upset and refused to eat anything. The rest of the party and the rest of the day were ruined. They didn't accept my apology. My comment hurt them too much. How could I have been so cruel?

Although not pencil thin, my daughters are far from having a weight problem. Libby would like to reduce the size of her hips, but basically she is comfortable with the size 10s and 12s she wears. Emily has a muscular physique (she's all athlete), but she, too, is fairly comfortable with her size.

If I continue to make these little digs (and I have made others before), I will drive both the girls straight to eating disorders. I know better! Why do I do this?

When I was a teenager (and probably even before), my mother thought she was helping me with her little comments about my weight. However, these comments only made me angry; the memory of them still does.

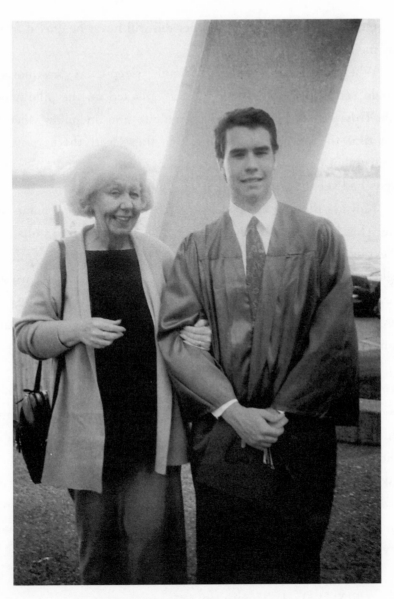

At Andrew's high school graduation.
We're so proud of each other.

One particular thing my mother did will never be erased from my memory. It was too hurtful.

Whenever I was invited to friends' sleep-overs, my mother would send me with a small "Crisco" marked on the pillowcase tab. This way, she said, I would be able to find my pillow when it was time to leave. (Keep in mind that these were the days when white pillowcases were the norm; designer sheets and fancy designs had yet to take over the linen industry.)

I always thought "Crisco" was my mom's endearing name for me. That is until I asked her the origin of the term. She smiled as she said, "It means 'fat in the can.'" I was so hurt. I couldn't believe she was so insensitive. I vowed at that time that I would never be so cruel if I ever had a daughter. However, maybe the saying "like mother, like daughter" is true. I was doing some of the same things to my daughters that my mother had done to me.

Happily, my mother has repented. She admits that she did not know the right way to help me. But I know the right way to help my daughters. And I know there is no excuse for saying weight things to them. I have to try harder to be more sensitive. If Libby and Emily want my help with their weight, I have to wait until they ask for it. I have to learn to keep my mouth shut. (These last words brought forth another bad memory. Before my mother was enlightened, she would say that there was only one thing wrong with me: my mouth. "Too much goes into it; too much comes out!")

WEDNESDAY, JUNE 18, 1997
What a day! A dream of a lifetime has come true! I sold my book, Slow But Sure . . . Now everyone will have the opportunity to follow in my weight-loss footsteps. Imagine! First I lost the weight—a great thing. Now I fulfilled another dream!

WEDNESDAY, JUNE 25, 1997

I continue to make some marvelous strides, literally. I've taken to walking just about everywhere. I walk daily to the health club (two and a half miles each way). I walk to friends' houses. (I used to drive half a block to visit my neighbor.) I walk half a mile to the school track, where I then walk another two or three miles.

A few weeks ago my husband and I decided to go out for dinner to our favorite Thai restaurant. (The owner accommodates my healthy eating and prepares my food in chicken broth instead of oil.) On this particular evening the weather was beautiful—sunny and in the comfortable seventies. "Let's walk," I said to Tom. He agreed. We did the almost-four-mile trek to the restaurant.

Tom and I continue to walk together on a regular basis. These escapes take us away from three noisy teenagers, the telephones (we have two lines that are always ringing), the television, and all the constant activity in our home. We walk and we talk. We spend quality time together.

MONDAY, JUNE 30, 1997

As the first six months of 1997 come to an end, I have decided that I'm not done with my weight-loss program. I have more than reached my goal. (Originally, I wanted to lose 150 pounds; I expanded my journey to 170 pounds!) Now I have decided that I would go a little farther down the road: Maybe another 10 pounds; maybe a little more. I won't do anything drastic—I will never do anything to affect my health—but I want to land in the 140s and at least give myself a 10-pound cushion.

While I have decided to lose a little more weight, I am also beginning to tackle maintenance. And I have discovered maintenance is not easy. The flood of graduation and other parties and

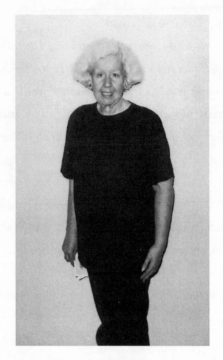

Summer 1997—152 pounds!

events that marked the last couple of months has shown me this. My weight fluctuated with all the food temptations. Luckily, I continued to focus on where I'd been; where I am; where I want to be. Because of this, I always get back to the 155 number on the scale. (I now weigh myself weekly on dreaded Mondays after food-filled weekends. This is a must to assure maintenance of the weight loss.)

I continue to be diligent. I have to be. Otherwise, I will find myself backtracking.

So now I'm working on a comfort cushion of at least 10 pounds. This is my new goal, my new journey. As before, I'll accomplish this passage with my proven slow but sure philosophy.

Chapter 13

Goodbye, Mrs. Claus!

In my sophomore year of college I had a crush on a fellow student whose last name was Closs. For weeks I spent extra time making sure my hair and nails were just perfect. (Because I was heavier than many of the other students, I concentrated on my best attributes. My nails were strong and long and my thick, naturally curly hair was, according to others, "fantastic.") I did my best to look my best. I was out to catch Mr. Closs.

My efforts and my "great sense of humor" (his words) attracted the intended prey. First, we went for coffee after class. Then we progressed to bona fide dates. I was in seventh heaven! Whoever said "a guy doesn't chat with a gal who is fat?"

After about two months of spending time together I opened my big mouth. Who knows what the conversation was about. All I remember is I said, "Just think. If we got married the preacher could end the ceremony with the words "I now pronounce you Sandy Closs." Instead of stopping there, I continued with "And then I would say, 'Ho! Ho! Ho!'" My Mr. Closs looked at me strangely. He didn't laugh. He immediately ended the date and took me home. I never heard from him again, just an occasional nod when we passed on campus.

Of course, I attributed this breakup to my weight. It had to be my weight! Nobody likes a fat girl. That's what years of thinking, reinforced by my mother's proclamations, had taught me. I never even considered that my attempt at humor scared him away.

Although I never became Mrs. Closs, on a number of occasions over the years small children asked me if I was Mrs. Claus. I did, after all, have white hair; I wore granny reading glasses, and I weighed more than 300 pounds. I couldn't blame the kids. I *did* have a resemblance to Santa's special spouse!

Now Mrs. Claus is gone. The white hair has been softened with an ash-blond toner and the bulging stomach has been replaced by firmed abs. The only remnant of the legendary Christmas Mrs. is the granny glasses. I still need them for reading.

With the exit of Mrs. Claus also came the withdrawal of some friends and family members. As I discovered early on my journey, overweight cohorts did not want me to leave them and trim ones didn't want me to join them. There are two clubs in this weight-conscious world and, I learned, it's hard to move from one to the other.

One friend is in the slender club. Over the years while she expressed concern about my weight, she treated me as if I were handicapped. When we went shopping together, she insisted upon loading all the groceries, hers and mine, into the car. I was verbally banished to the passenger's seat. I wasn't allowed to help. It was, according to her, easier for her to do it. When our families vacationed together, she insisted on doing all the cleaning and cooking. Again, according to her, it was easier for her to do it.

I recently realized that her assistance in years past was her way of feeling better than me. It gave her a sense of superiority. Now I am the same weight as this "friend." However, physically, I'm more fit and I have more energy than she does. (I exercise daily; she doesn't.) I no longer allow her to wait on me. She doesn't like this. She wants "poor impaired Sandy" back in her life. She says I've changed, and I have, but the changes aren't with the inside me, only the outside. And the new outside allows me to do things for myself. I've lost weight and, because of this, I've also lost a friend.

As sad as it is to lose a friend, losing a close family member has been particularly painful. This family member is in the other club—the one consisting of overweight members. Now, because of 170 pounds, I've lost my membership! And, like the majority of the members in this organization, this family member doesn't want to have anything to do with me. I'm not her "fat buddy" anymore. I never thought that weight would come between us, but it has. My success only serves to remind her of her failure in the weight-loss game. Because of this, our relationship is almost nonexistent, and I miss her. However, I've done what I needed to do for my health. And, whenever she is ready, I'll be there to help her. Hopefully, some semblance of a relationship will return slowly but surely. Hopefully, she will get used to my new outer covering and realize I'm still me!

Many of my relationships have changed with the weight loss. When I started this journey, I thought everyone would be happy for me when I reached my goal. I never thought there would be a negative side to such a positive accomplishment. Boy, was I wrong!

Although saddened by the lack of positive response I've received from some, I've had mostly praise from Tom and the kids. I say "mostly" because they, too, are having problems adjusting to their new wife and mother.

Tom tells me daily how proud he is of me. However, some of

his other words reveal that he is not totally secure with my weight loss.

"Now that you're skinny, you're not going to leave me, are you?" he has asked a few times. (As I've previously stated, in the past during heated arguments, I've threatened this. Tom apparently took me seriously!)

"Are you meeting your boyfriend?" Tom has asked when I leave the house for nightly walks or workouts at the health club. (He never asked this when I was heavy. Then again, I rarely went out at night in my pre-exercise days.)

I now spend a great deal of time reassuring the man I married that the only thing that has changed is my body.

"My love for you is just as strong as—if not stronger than—when I was overweight," I tell him. I remind him of his complete acceptance of me when I was obese . . . of how he always treated me as if I were beautiful, no matter what my size. Also, I tell him that my success is due, in large part, to his support, encouragement, and his firm belief that I would reach my goal.

"I lost weight so we can be together longer and more fully," I tell him. "I want to be the best I can be for myself and for you and the kids. I love you deeply and this will never change."

These words are reinforced with lots of hugs and kisses and even my initiation of sex. (Boy! Have I come a long way!) Hopefully, with time, these efforts will boost his confidence.

As much as Tom and I are working to assure that our relationship remains strong amid the changes that have resulted from my weight loss, there are times of marital difficulty. I have become less tolerant of my husband's imperfections. I feel that if I have done this "great thing," Tom should be able to change some little things, such as his poor eating habits. He promises often; he rarely delivers. While I now make healthy meals, he continues to down peanut butter or bologna sandwiches (lots) for dinner. He avoids fruits and vegetables and fills up instead on potato chips.

Tom does not have a weight problem (all his adult life he's been in the 160–170-pound range) and he's active (in addition to being an engineer, he's also a basketball official and spends many hours on weeknights and weekends running the courts), but this doesn't mean he's healthy. We recently discovered that he has high blood pressure requiring medication. I know (as does he) that his diet has a lot to do with this medical condition. But has he changed his poor eating habits? No! And this has been the source of numerous spats. Four years ago he feared for my life; now I fear for his!

Another fear of mine is that my golden years will find me in good health and eager to enjoy life, but forced to push my husband around in a wheelchair or, even worse, confined to the home to provide him with constant nursing.

Every time I see Tom scarfing down unhealthy foods, I cringe. I resent what he is doing to himself. If I loved him enough to lose weight in order to improve our life together, why can't he make some dietary adjustments?

Wait a second! I, of all people, know that nobody can be pushed into action. A person has to reach a point where enough is enough. An individual has to decide for him- or herself to take the steps necessary for success. Doctors and a screaming spouse aren't going to get Tom to this point unless that's where he wants to be. I have to keep quiet, set a good example, and pray. Hopefully, Tom will soon begin to make the changes needed to assure long life and good health. He's promised!

While Tom and others are adjusting to the new me, my children have readily accepted their slim, healthy mom. Of course, they are the same individuals who looked at me lovingly over the years when I was fat (and wore a bathing suit), when my hair was dirty, when I hadn't yet brushed my teeth or taken a shower, when my clothes didn't match, and all the other times when I wasn't perfect. I guess what I'm saying is that my kids just accept me any way I am. For better or worse, I'm just their mom.

However, while the kids like my new look, it has put some pressure on them—especially the girls. Teenage girls as a group tend to be overly concerned about weight. Libby and Emily seemed to have skipped this phase . . . that is, until I lost my excess weight. Now they look at me each and every time they put food on their plates; take a cookie or two out of the jar; have a dish of ice cream. They seem to be waiting for me to say something (at times I have)!

There is a discomfort level not only with food, but also with the fact that we can wear many of the same size clothes. How can this be! When they were small girls I had to get old clothes from trim friends so they could play "dress up." Mine were way too large. Now I am wearing clothes their size. They're used to me being their fat mom (although they never verbalized this; it's just the way it was), and so they have falsely rationalized that if they're wearing the same size clothes as Mom, they must be fat!

Lots of talks and sharing of feelings is helping us understand each other. I try to keep my mouth shut when I see them make poor but "teenage normal" food choices. I invite them to walk and work out with me, which they do if their busy schedules allow. And I stay out of their closets (something I wish they would do in my room)!

These efforts are making a difference. The girls are getting used to my size and I'm being more sensitive to their concerns. But it does take work, the mental variety!

Work! I never anticipated that there would be this much work at the end of the journey. I thought everyone would be happy for me . . . would revel in my success. I thought everything would be wonderful!

Okay! So everything's not wonderful. I can live with that. What I'm having a real problem with is trying to discover who I am. Some days I just don't know.

I'm a wife. I'm a mother. I'm a sister, a daughter, a friend. However—and here's the hard part—if I'm no longer the fat lady, who am I?

I'm where I always wanted to be, where I always dreamed I'd be—healthy and trim—but it's taking time and effort to adjust to this new place. My head hasn't caught up with the body. I still feel fat, and, because of this, I shy away from compliments. I want to say "no big deal" when I'm told how good I look.

So why isn't it a big deal to me? I feel somewhat ashamed that I got so fat in the first place. I feel that I shouldn't be rewarded with praise for something I should have done years ago. Others have done great things, overcome great obstacles. All I did was begin to eat healthy and exercise on a regular basis. This is something I should have been doing anyway.

When I was a small child, my mother taught me to just say "thank you" when someone extended a compliment. If someone said, "What a pretty dress," I was taught to refrain from saying such things as "It was really cheap!" or "This old thing!" or "I bought it at the secondhand store!" According to Mom, I should "just say thank you and leave it at that!" So I try, and sometimes it's really hard, especially when people use "skinny" in their compliments, to just say "thank you." In my mind, these compliment-givers are nuts!

I also think some of the men I know are nuts. That's because they have taken to flirting with me. Imagine! Men are flirting with me! These are the very same individuals who just a few years ago treated me as their buddy. Now they act as if I'm a budding sex symbol. And I'm not comfortable with this role. (Neither are their wives!)

I ward off this unwanted attention with humor and I stay away from making off-color comments. (Before we shared jokes, even "dirty" jokes. Now this isn't possible.) Also, I sprinkle "Tom" and "the kids" throughout my conversations with members of the opposite sex. And I act naïve and play dumb. It works.

So who am I? Am I the skinny, sexy woman of Beverly Hills, Michigan? I don't think so! But I'm also not one of the largest women in my ten thousand–plus community. I guess I'm somewhere in between. And it's going to take some time to get used to this new place! But I'll do it! (And I will stay here! I will not be one of the 90 or so percent of dieters who gain back their weight!)

Slowly but surely, I'll become comfortable with this new place, as will my family and friends. It *is* a nice place to be . . . and with a little effort on their part, they can join me. I'd like that!

Be Realistic!

- Don't expect that everyone will be happy with your weight-loss success. Fewer pounds can and often do spur jealousy in others, especially those with weight problems.
- Don't expect acceptance of the new you immediately. It's going to take time for you and others to become comfortable with your size. The slow but sure approach that helped you with the weight loss can aid in acceptance, too.
- Don't expect your life to change drastically when you

lose weight. Problems (except maybe those stemming from health) that you had before the weight loss will not automatically disappear. You'll just be in better shape to handle them.

- Don't expect others to like you better because you weigh less. If you were likable and lovable before you lost weight—and you keep your success in perspective (no boasting . . . no arrogance)—you'll still be likable and lovable. If you weren't so nice, this is your next challenge!

- Don't expect maintenance to be easy. You need the same efforts (exercise and a healthy food plan) that resulted in weight loss to keep the weight off. Lessen these efforts and the pounds will return.

- Don't expect that you can go it alone now that you're fit and trim. Continue to seek God's help. Everyday living and food temptations will always be difficult. However, God will help. Just ask Him!

Chapter 14

A Happy Medium!

Twenty-five years ago I ended an engagement with a horticul-
turalist whose hobby was to create oil paintings of dead flow-
ers and foliage. (Now, if that wasn't a clue that something was
wrong with this man, nothing was!) Also, our only shared interest
was food. About the only thing we did together was eat. And the
only growth we shared was our body size.

At the time of our breakup, I was living with this plant man
(tsk! tsk!), away from family and friends. (He was getting an ad-
vanced degree at a college in another part of the state.) Once I
removed him from the premises, I needed something to fill the
time after work. I found a fortune-teller and began taking lessons
in card reading from her, especially since I always thought I had
some psychic powers. The fortune teller agreed. (It was still another thing I could do in a seated position.) I became a medium
("Madame SaSu"—from *Sandra Sue*), but I wasn't happy.

Now I'm a happy medium. I no longer wear large or extra large
or plus-size clothing. I wear medium. There is joy in my heart

when I walk into clothing stores and head for the medium racks. I'm no longer too big and I'm not too small. I'm just right. I'm a medium!

(By the way. Madame SaSu is no more. I don't have time to sit around. I'm too busy exercising and enjoying life. Besides, I believe God is the only way to the future . . . God and our own good efforts!)

TUESDAY–WEDNESDAY, JULY 22–23, 1997

Parents' orientation at Michigan State University. I went alone because Tom couldn't get off work. Soon after I arrived I met another parent—a man—in the elevator. We were on our way to lunch and decided to sit together. We ended up spending the two days together—all meals and free time. Nothing happened but friendship. A good Christian man, he talked about his spouse and three children. A good Christian woman, I did the same. However, these meetings made me feel—for one of the few times in my life—like an attractive woman. I felt comfortable without the embarrassment of excess weight. Also, on Tuesday night, we decided to do a healthy four-mile walk around campus. I set the pace and my trim friend had a problem, at times, keeping up with me. How exhilarating!

THURSDAY, AUGUST 22, 1997

Today was a particularly difficult day. I drove my firstborn to college. This just came too fast. I like having all my little chicks in the nest. Now there will be an empty space.

Before we left, Andy picked me up, literally. After all those years of picking up my son, first as a baby, then as a toddler, my son is now able to pick me up. My weight is no longer a problem. Andy picked me up to tell me thank you for everything I had done for him as his mother. It was a special and tearful moment for us both.

MONDAY, SEPTEMBER 1, 1997

My best friend, Marilyn Dailey, and I decided to mix getting together and fitness with good causes. We signed up for six-mile walks with our entry fees going to charities. What a healthy way to make time in our busy schedules to see one another.

TUESDAY, SEPTEMBER 9, 1997

I fell down on the sidewalk today during one of my power walks. My right knee swelled to five times its normal size and the whole right side of my body is severely bruised. As much as I am in pain, I am even more upset because this accident will curtail my exercise. I now love to exercise (There! I've said it!) and I especially like to walk out-of-doors.

SUNDAY, SEPTEMBER 28, 1997

Boy! Can I be stupid at times! Marilyn and I had planned to partici-pate in the Gilda (Radner) Walk, so, knee injury and all, I walked the six miles. (This was especially important because a friend of mine is currently fighting ovarian cancer, the disease that took the life of the comedian for whom this event is named.) Needless to say, the walk took its toll on my knee. Stupid! Stupid! Stupid!

OCTOBER–DECEMBER 1997

Depression hit big time during the final months of the year. My knee continued to be a problem and my arm, which also took the impact of the fall, was in constant pain from a hairline fracture and tendon damage. I was forced to refrain from exercise and because of this, I became depressed. I fed my depression with sweets, and some pounds (I'm not sure how many—I was afraid to get on the scale) crept onto my body.

One day near year's end when I was particularly upset, I pur-

chased six large chocolate eclairs for comfort. Just as I was about to bite into the first one, the phone rang. It was Richard Simmons. A few soothing words from him about my great success and how far I'd come led to a nice treat for the garbage disposal. How did he know?

JANUARY 1998

I can exercise again. Thank heavens. The inactivity and the holidays took a toll. I have gained 15 pounds and am back up to 170. But I'm not worried. Exercise and attention to my food plan will get it off. Then I'll work toward my new goal of 144. (I was born in 1944 so weighing 144 pounds just seems right for me. I'm just glad I wasn't born in 1922!) I'm back on the move . . . I'm back on the road!

VALENTINE'S DAY, FEBRUARY 14, 1998

Some years ago, a book entitled The Total Woman *was a bestseller. One suggestion in the book was to greet your husband at the door enrobed only in plastic wrap. I remember thinking at the time that a roll of this wrapping probably would not be long enough to go around my ample body. I also decided that "clear" definitely wasn't my color. However, I did think the suggestion had some merit for keeping the home fires burning. Now was the time to put this suggestion into action. What a great Valentine's treat for my husband.*

All three of the children were gone, an extremely rare occurrence. Andy was at college; the girls were on school trips. It was definitely time for the plastic wrap, especially since my body is smaller and this covering now comes in colors. I chose "rose crystal." It's definitely me!

My husband was expected home at 7:30 P.M. At 7:15 I began wrapping. Although shivering (it was, after all, winter in Michigan) and sweating (that's what plastic does to your skin) at the same time, I was ready for my man. The appointed time came and went. So did

8 *P.M.*, 8:30 *P.M.*, 9 *P.M.* I worried that my husband was in an accident and I would scare away the police if they came to the door with the news. Then the phone rang.

"I had to fill in for a couple of basketball games," said my husband, the referee. "I'm sorry, but I didn't have time to call you."

He was really sorry when I told him what I was wearing and what I had in mind. He groaned.

Tom is still groaning about his missed opportunity. I reminded him that it will probably be four years until we're alone again. That's when our youngest goes off to college.

WEDNESDAY, MARCH 11, 1998

Where I was came back to me today when I spoke to a group of women who weigh 300 or more pounds. I watched how they walked with effort. I saw the pain in their eyes and heard it in their words when they told me of health problems resulting from the excess weight. I told my story; offered encouragement and hope. However, to my dismay, these women were filled with excuses. They wanted a magic solution that didn't require much effort on their part. This was a sobering experience. I had been there!

I vowed today that I'll never get heavy again . . . especially now that I'm almost back to the 155-pound mark. I like good health. I like being fit. I like being smaller!

THURSDAY, MARCH 12, 1998

A sad, sad day. A good friend of many years was diagnosed with brain and lung cancer. We used to sneak out of school functions and smoke together. Lately, I've been sneaking cigarettes from her. No more! No more! Especially since my occasional cigarettes are becoming more than occasional. I promised her; I promised myself. No more!

THURSDAY, MARCH 19, 1998

Spoke to more than one hundred senior high school students on the importance of fitness. They were very receptive to me and my words. Losing weight and getting fit have enabled me to motivate others. What a positive mark I am making!

SATURDAY, MARCH 28, 1998

Went shopping for spring/summer clothes. One of the nicest things about losing weight is that I no longer have to constantly tug my tops down over my hips to hide the enormity of my rear. Also, no longer do I have to keep my coat on at all times to hide my body. I now buy body-fitting clothes because my body is fit!

MONTH OF APRIL 1998

Walking, working out, and writing. These wonderful activities mark the month as spring makes its appearance in Michigan. My girls have followed my lead and work out together every night at the health club. Libby, since January, has shed more than 10 pounds. Athletic Emily has dropped 5. How fit they both are. Fit and lovely!

FRIDAY, MAY 15, 1998

The battle of the bulge is an ongoing challenge. I'm totally cigarette-free (and crabby) and I've added a few pounds. I've increased my exercise (three-mile walks in the morning, two-mile walks in the evening, and one hour daily of aerobics and/or toning and abs work at the health club). Also, I'm being more diligent (again) about what goes into my mouth. Will it ever end? I, of all people, know the answer to this. Fitness and healthy eating require a lifelong commitment. Alas! I'm back down to 155 pounds. I did it!

MEMORIAL DAY WEEKEND, 1998

Three parties and three events offering smoking and eating tempta-
tions. I did well on both fronts. I'm on that road to my new 144-
pound goal. No more side trips! The only way I'll do it is by sticking
to the straight and narrow. *(Now there's a good word!)*

Chapter 15

Heavy Thoughts on the Lighter Side!

When you go on a journey such as mine, you pick up all sorts of souvenirs along the way. Instead of putting these keepsakes in a memory box or stashing them in some drawer, I want to share mine with you. I also like to keep them out for myself. They remind me of where I've been and help keep me at my destination.

Oops! Sometimes I goof. And you, too, will have setbacks if you don't watch out for the following pitfalls:

- *Skipping meals.* You need to eat three meals a day at suitably spaced intervals to be sure you have enough energy and so that hunger won't overwhelm you. Skip breakfast and you'll tend to eat more at lunch; skip lunch and, chances are, you'll overdo at dinner; skip dinner and you'll probably find yourself gorging on snacks at night.

- *Overeating at get-togethers, special occasions, and on weekends.* These are my biggest challenges and, most likely, yours, too! It's hard to stay on your food plan when confronted by the temptations these events offer, but it can be done. All it takes is determination and a mental plan to stay away from the food table. Prepare for the event with a full stomach (have a veggie salad or veggie soup before you leave the house) and don't even look at the food when you arrive.

- *Eating when bored or stressed.* I clean my closets when I'm bored; I work out when I'm stressed. Finding an enjoyable or useful activity instead of turning to food can alleviate boredom and stress.

- *Not drinking enough fluids, especially water.* Many times when we think we're hungry, we're just thirsty. Drinking a glass of water can help us stay away from unplanned eating. Remember, there are no calories in water!

Imagine a world where everybody is the perfect size, a world where tall people are slender; short people are trim. Think you would like such a world? If you're overweight and dream of being your perfect size, you might be tempted to answer yes! But think about it. Wouldn't this perfect world be especially dull, at least visually?

Visualize a beautifully decorated Christmas tree. Now look at the presents beneath this tree. Imagine that they are all superbly wrapped and all the same size. Are you excited about opening these presents? Probably not! There's no intriguing variety. Everything is the same.

Compare yourself to a present under a Christmas tree, a regular tree in our real world. You may be large; you may be small. You may be exquisitely wrapped; you may just have a bow stuck on top of dime-store paper. However, what this mental picture does offer is variety on the outside, and interest in what's on the inside.

When we are overweight, we tend to concentrate so much on the flaws of our package that we forget to consider the special gift inside. We overlook the uniqueness of who we are and how much we add to the picture of life.

Before you try to change your outer package, you must learn to appreciate what you have inside. You need to realize that each and every one of us is a special gift.

Once you realize your specialness and appreciate all that you have to offer, you'll be able to work on the wrapping. You need not strive for perfection, just work toward improving the package. You can be one of the most precious presents under the Christmas tree, but only if you believe it's what's inside that counts!

While on your journey to weight loss and fitness wear outfits in a single color. Clothing, stockings, and shoes, all the same color, can give you a sleek, smooth appearance.

For years, like many good mothers, I made cookies, especially chocolate chip, for the kids. The recipe I used stated a yield of three dozen cookies. I never got more than two dozen.

My daughters are now the family's cookie makers. They are amazed at how many cookies they get from the very same recipe. They get the promised three dozen.

I used to eat a dozen "cookies" before I even baked the batter. I used to "test" each recipe by eating a hearty serving while I cooked. I used to nibble slices of luncheon meat while I made the kids' lunches. And, as I was doing this, I expressed dismay over my increasing weight. "I don't eat that much," I told the doctor as the scale kept going up. Who was I kidding?

To get a laugh, I used to tell people, "If you are what you eat, why am I not tall and slender like a Twinkie?" Now I truly am what I eat! I'm sort of tall—5'7"—and slender like a celery stalk, or, more realistically, like a carrot, with a few bumps here and there!

I think it's important for you to realize that although your life may change physically when you lose weight, who you truly are will not drastically change. If people liked and accepted you before you lost weight, they'll like and accept you at a smaller size. The reverse is also true.

Years ago I worked with a woman who wasn't a very pleasant person. She was always negative and critical of others. She had problems making and keeping friends. She decided to lose weight. She thought her weight was keeping her from successful relationships, of both the male and female variety.

She lost a tremendous amount of weight over a two-year period. Her former fat, dumpy self was transformed into a stunning woman. She prepared herself with clothes and makeup for an onslaught of men. And she thought that everyone would like her better because she was thin. It didn't happen because she was still the same negative, critical person she had always been.

In less than a year, this woman gained back the weight she had lost and then some. She was bitter and became even less pleasant to be around.

Losing weight isn't the solution to all the problems in your life.

It is a solution for achieving good health and fitness. However, other aspects of your life should be evaluated and, if necessary, altered to achieve your very best you.

When I was overweight I'd tell people I was on a "seafood" diet. "Whenever I *see* food, I eat it!" This brought laughs.

Now I've learned that "out of sight, out of mind" is a better approach. I stopped putting the kids' cookies in my clear cookie jar (it now contains packages of low-fat popcorn), and the candy dishes go unfilled. Unhealthy treats are now less available, hidden in their packages and stored in rarely used cupboards.

Three steps were especially beneficial when I started my journey. These steps could also lead you to success.

- *Stop dieting.* Instead, develop your own healthy food plan of moderation and balance based on a sensible caloric intake.

- *Start by making small changes.* Replace your afternoon candy bar with a small apple. Cut the amount of spaghetti you eat in half. Order less-fattening seafood when you dine out instead of your normal steak. Replace whole milk with skim milk. Eat half of a small banana instead of a large whole one.

- *Don't expect miracles.* You've spent years in an unhealthy eating mode. You can't expect perfection immediately—or ever. Just try to do better about making healthy food choices, and add regular exercise to your

life. If you goof (which we all do), try again and keep
trying.

I conquered my weight one meal at a time . . . one day at a
time . . . one pound at a time. I found that anything more was
unrealistic. At times I would get discouraged when I lost *only* a
pound. Then I would go to the meat section of the grocery store
and pick up and look at a pound of hamburger. This is what I lost!
It reminded me that I was making progress. I especially loved those
days when I was able to pick up a family pack of five pounds or
more of hamburger!

So you're on a plateau and you want to push the scale down a
notch. A *moderate* calorie reduction is more effective than taking
drastic measures. You might want to cut a starch (bread, pasta,
potato) or two out of your daily food plan. Or eat one less protein.
But don't cut your dairy servings (you need the calcium) or your
fruits and vegetables.

All you need to achieve physical fitness is thirty minutes (This can
be done throughout the day in three ten-minute sessions) of moderate physical activity, such as brisk walking, seven days a week. If
you want to lose weight, you may need to exercise longer or at a
greater intensity.

I exercise each and every day at the Beverly Hills Racquet and
Health Club, which is two miles from my home. On most nice
days I leave my car at home and walk the two miles there and back.
(I've even done this in a snowstorm and in frigid weather when my
car wouldn't start. I didn't want to miss exercising!)

Across from the club is a cemetery. Each day when I come out of the club I face the cemetery. This serves to remind me that if I don't keep coming to the right side of the road, I'll end up too soon on the wrong side.

When my kids were small and all the other mothers were teaching their children the ABCs, I taught mine the vowels—"A, E, I, O, U, and sometimes Y." When those other mothers proudly had their little stars dutifully recite the alphabet to show off their exceptional knowledge, I'd listen and offer praise. "That's great," I'd say, "but my child knows the vowels!" Then the Prysby child being showcased would enthusiastically spit out "A, E, I, O, U, and sometimes Y." The mothers were impressed. They thought my child had superior intelligence.

This stunt was fun, but it didn't eliminate the need to teach my children their ABCs. The kids still had to be ready to meet their peers in pre-school.

Diets are like teaching your kids "just the vowels." They are temporary fixes, little tricks, shortcuts that help you lose the 20 pounds by such-and-such a date. However, diets aren't lasting, nor is the resultant weight loss. The pounds almost always come back.

You need the whole alphabet. You need to learn to change your lifestyle to assure permanent success.

An Alphabet for Success!

A — **Avoid negative thoughts and add positive, optimistic people to your life.**

B — **Believe in yourself. Know that you are capable of achieving your goals.**

C — Control your desire to go too fast and concentrate on a slow but sure approach.

D — Design a balanced food plan filled with lots of fruits and vegetables.

E — Exercise regularly. It's the only way to achieve physical fitness.

F — Focus on your successes, no matter how small; not on your mistakes.

G — Give yourself permission to be human. Be kind to yourself when you have difficulty on the journey.

H — Help yourself succeed by taking the time to plan and prepare good food and to exercise.

I — Invest in a food scale and use it daily to keep portion sizes in check, and a scale (used sparingly) to check on your weight and your progress.

J — Join up with others on the same road for support.

K — Keep a food diary. Experts say this is one of the best ways to lose weight successfully.

L — Lift your spirit and renew your determination with a few minutes of quiet reflection each day.

M — Make each day count. Each morning vow to do well and work toward this mini-goal.

N — Nurture yourself with treats such as a bubble bath, a favorite song, a good book.

O — Obtain the support of family and friends. This can make all the difference!

P — Plan . . . plan . . . plan. It is only through planning (food and exercise) that you can succeed!

Q — Quell temptations by keeping healthy foods on hand.

R — Rely on your inner strength and God. You've got what it takes and God will help you.

S — Savor your success, no matter how small.

T — Take charge. Don't let anyone or anything keep you from your goals.

U — Understand that you're not perfect. Know this and you'll do perfectly fine!

V — Vary your exercise. Doing the same thing every day is good, but mixing it up is better!

W — Water yourself! H_2O and lots of it works . . . on your body, your skin, your weight loss!

X — X out bad feelings about yourself and bad foods for your body.

Y — Yearn for success. A passionate zeal for a healthier life can move you to action.

Z — Zip your lips when faced with unhealthy food choices and you'll zap the craving in twenty minutes or less!

Just think! The word "thin" makes up most of the word "think." I guess this means that in order to be thin, we have to think about it. We have to think about what we put in our mouths; we have to think about putting exercise in our lives.

• • •

Why do fast-food chains, especially those that serve extremely high-fat fare, fail to accommodate fat patrons?

I never used to fit comfortably into the booths at fast-food restaurants. I'd have to squeeze myself into the seats, so much so that I would bruise my abdomen. I'd do this because I didn't want to embarrass my children. I didn't want them to think that their mom was too fat to be in public. I wanted them to think they had a regular mom.

Now I can fit into any seat or any booth, and usually with room to spare. This is another small measure of success. However, now that I fit, I rarely patronize fast-food restaurants. When I do go, I select foods that fit into my healthy eating plan!

Since I've lost weight, my fingers look and feel like sticks. I like to clasp my fingers together and feel their slenderness. When I get discouraged—which sometimes I still do—I put my hands together, then intertwine my fingers. It's my own personal reminder of success. It works even better than looking into a mirror. Often, while my fingers are entwined, I take time to thank God for all His help.

For years I hadn't been able to kneel on the kneelers in church. My body was just too big. However, now my body is small enough to fit in the space comfortably, and my knees are strong enough to support my weight. How far I've come. Now I'm kneeling in church. I think God is happy. I know I am!

A reminder from Richard Simmons: "I know you want to help the world, Sandy, and I think you are helping so many. You know what it's like to catch the bug and you want to spread it to everyone. However, you know as well as I, until you're ready to do this thing, it just never happens."

"Slow and steady

wins the race."

—The Hare and

the Tortoise,

AESOP,

550 B.C.